IF I COULD JUST SNAP OUT OF IT, DON'T YOU THINK I WOULD?

A NINE-MONTH PLAN FOR SMASHING YOUR DEPRESSION

by
Cathy Goldstein Mullin, MSW, LICSW

Copyright © 2012 by Cathy Goldstein Mullin, LICSW

All rights reserved. Except as indicated, no part of this book may be reproduced, translated, stored in a retrieval system, or transmitted, in any form or by any means, electronic, mechanical, photocopying, microfilming, recording or otherwise, without written permission of the author.

Limited Photocopy License
The author grants to individual purchasers of this book non-assignable permission to reproduce the forms and calendar in this book for personal use. This license is limited to the purchasers of this book for personal use or for therapeutic use with clients. This license does not grant the right to reproduce the material within this book for resale, redistribution, or any other purpose.

Copyediting by David Downer

First published by Dog Ear Publishing
4010 W. 86th Street, Ste H
Indianapolis, IN 46268
www.dogearpublishing.net

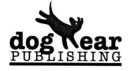

ISBN: 978-1-4575-0890-5

This book is printed on acid-free paper.

Printed in the United States of America

DEDICATED TO MY FATHER, SIDNEY ALAN GOLDSTEIN, WHO TOLD ME THAT THE BEST WAY TO BEAT DEPRESSION WAS TO STAY BUSY AND EAT BRAN, AND TO MY TWO WONDERFUL CHILDREN, ALEXA AND SAMANTHA, WHO TAUGHT ME THAT THE MORE ONE WORKS AT LIFE, THE RICHER IT GETS.

ACKNOWLEDGMENTS

I have learned almost all of what I know about depression from my clients–kids, adolescents, and adults who have been willing to share their dark days and bleak thoughts. No matter how bad things got for them, most were willing to take very deep breaths and do the really hard work necessary to get better.

Also, I want to thank the clinical staff at MassGeneral for Children at North Shore Medical Center in Salem, Massachusetts for creating an environment where learning flourishes and baring the soul is considered a true act of courage.

TABLE OF CONTENTS

CHAPTER ONE	I HATE MY DEPRESSION	1
CHAPTER TWO	WHAT THIS BOOK OFFERS	6
CHAPTER THREE	WHEN MEDICATION COMES FIRST	20
CHAPTER FOUR	FACING YOUR ANGER	...27
CHAPTER FIVE	ONE, TWO, THREE AND THE DAMAGE IS DONE	..37
CHAPTER SIX	REACHING YOUR GOALS	48
CHAPTER SEVEN	WEAR YOUR COGNITIVE HAT	64
CHAPTER EIGHT	CHANGING YOUR BEHAVIOR	92
CHAPTER NINE	CHOOSING FROM THE B LIST	116

CHAPTER TEN   HURDLES 145

CHAPTER ELEVEN   TYING IT ALL
                 TOGETHER 150

CHAPTER ONE

I HATE MY DEPRESSION

O.K. SAY IT. LIFE stinks.
Too Pollyanna-like for you? O. K., then. Life sucks.
You're depressed. Always depressed. Nothing's fun anymore. You can't remember when it was.
School, jobs-these are just things you have to do.
Money-there's something there's never enough of.
Love. That's a joke-some fantasy somebody made up to keep all the fools going.
You hate feeling depressed. Who wouldn't? But you didn't choose it.
It's not like you said, "Hey, depression, come over here. I want to hang out with you." It's just how you feel. You've been depressed for so long, you can't remember being anything else. Maybe it's part of your genes.
O.K., well, maybe it is. But what are you going to do about it?
"What do you mean, 'What am I going to do about it?'"
Let me make an analogy. Suppose you went for a physical and learned you had cancer. If you are anything like me, hysteria would immediately take over. After a day of sobs, the plea bargaining would begin. "Please God, if you let me get through this, I'll change my ways. I'll be nicer. I'll appreciate things more. I'll quit smoking. I'll be a better parent."
As the days passed and the sheer terror abated, you'd berate the universe. "It's not fair. Why me? What the hell have I ever done?" Eventually, though, you'd put the doom, gloom, and pity aside and go about the very serious business of making decisions. You'd meet with your doctors, your

family. You'd consider chemotherapy, radiation. You'd know that what lay ahead would be brutally difficult. But you'd go forth with the treatment anyway, because you'd know you'd be fighting for your life.

It's the same with depression.

"But cancer's an illness," you say. "Depression is different. It's just me."

I've got news for you. Your brain's a part of your body-just another organ. More sophisticated, yes, but another organ. And when your brain's chemistry doesn't work right, it is as much an illness as when your liver cells mess up. And it requires just as much of a fight.

"But I don't want to fight my depression. I just want it to go away."

O.K., I get it. You can't be blamed for wanting it to be easier. It's the way of our world—a world where our every question can be answered instantaneously in cyberspace, where a click of a switch offers make-believe fire, where the virtual world is the biggest shopping mall there is, and where email trumps the postal service every day of the week.

Yes. Technology has changed our lives and made things easier. But it hasn't taught us to fight the big stuff.

If I Could Just Snap Out of It, Don't You Think I Would? is a book about doing something big about your depression. It's a book about making a serious commitment to improving the quality of your life. People with depression can get better if they work at it. Sure, they may have flare-ups in their lives, flare-ups that people without depression may not have. But so what? They can go on to live full, rich lives.

But you can't get better if you don't work at it. Just like the person with cancer may not be alive five years from now if she doesn't fight.

That's what this book is about-it's about fighting for your life. Fighting to have a big slice of the happiness pie. If you are willing to fight your depression, to fight really hard, keep reading. If you insist that your depression just disappear instantly—with a press of a button or a snap of your fingers—throw this book away.

WHAT CAUSES DEPRESSION?

Genes are responsible for some depression. Simply put, if granddaddy was depressed, daddy bipolar, and mom sad and obsessive, you may have inherited the predisposition to depression from all of them. It is as if some people are the unlucky winners of their clan's depressive gene lottery.

Genes also help determine our brain chemistry. Our brains function using chemicals whose primary task is to ensure that we can send, receive, and interpret messages. These same chemicals also tell us how to feel about the messages we receive. It is known there is a relationship between brain chemistry and depression.

Say we awaken on a Saturday to a sunny, warm day and blue skies. First, our brain has to determine that beautiful sunshine, warm temperatures, and blue skies equal good weather as opposed to tumultuous weather or plain nasty weather, and good weather means that we can go outside and enjoy the day. Then our brain has to run through its menu of things we enjoy doing on beautiful, warm, weekend days. A well-functioning brain will typically experience pleasure at the thought of engaging in a pleasant, warm-weather activity, thus suggesting to us that it would be a good idea to choose a similar, fun activity for today. This thought would then cause us to experience happiness, resulting in messages being sent from our brain, causing us to move our feet onto the floor, jump up, and begin the day.

A brain without the proper mix of chemicals, however, may not experience pleasure at the thought of engaging in what was once a fun activity. Because we don't experience pleasure at this thought, our brain doesn't instruct us to get moving. Rather, our brain goes into slow-down mode and instructs us to scoot our hips backward and crawl back under the covers.

Those who inherit depression from their families often have trouble finding pleasure in any activity. But ask them to list the negatives and the answers come quickly.

Yes, sometimes, the brain chemistry we inherit is askew. Other times, it's family life that does us in.

Kids are at the mercy of their parents or caretakers. When these people are cruel, kids suffer.

"You're a chicken-shit faggot," a father says to his son. "On second thought, chickens have more balls."

"Get used to working on your knees. That's all you are good for," says a mother to her daughter.

"You're stupid," says a father to his child. "Lazy and stupid."

"Stop eating. You eat like a pig," says a mother to her son.

These are actual statements made to clients by their caretakers. The recipients, now grown men and women, have been in therapy for years. Their issue is self-esteem and the work required for them to heal has been tremendous.

Alcoholic and/or drug-addicted caretakers also wreak havoc on their kids.

I will never forget the story of my client's father, a severe and miserable alcoholic, who threw my client, then seven years old, into a Louisiana swamp filled with crocodiles. The father thought it was funny. If it hadn't been for the father's girlfriend, who happened to be sober that night, the boy would not have been around to tell his story. But the damage done to this boy, now a man, has lasted a lifetime.

Ditto for the damage done to children used for sex. Without a great deal of work, children who are sexually exploited grow into adults whose spirits are deadened and souls destroyed. And even though adults who have been abused go to great lengths to dull the memories and quiet the voices so they don't have to remember, the memories often come anyway.

"Uncle Robert loves you the best," they hear their uncles, neighbors, club leaders saying. "That's why we're doing this.

But you can't tell anyone, because they won't understand how much we love each other."

Depression has various origins. But where it comes from doesn't matter. What matters is what we do with it.

CHAPTER TWO
WHAT THIS BOOK OFFERS

FOR THE LAST TWELVE YEARS I have been a therapist, working with kids, teenagers, and adults. My clients are wonderful people. Many of them have depression. Some have cut, slicing their arms like so many cucumbers; others have attempted suicide. Some have no family or friends, others are surrounded by family. Some are jobless and housebound. Some have full-time jobs.

What all these people have in common is a sense of being beaten by their depression, of being helpless against the monster of their disorder. The majority of my clients have tried to fight. Many feel they have failed.

I've worked with some of these people for months, others for years. But what is consistent is that they arrive for their therapy sessions at least once a month, discouraged. Together we sit, putting the pieces back together, restoring their hopes.

They leave excited, determined.

But the gains seldom last.

I had to ask myself some tough questions. Why were my clients finding it so hard to fight their depression? Why didn't they finish their weekly assignments when they understood the sense of the assignments when in session? Why were they giving up?

I came to see that fighting depression is a herculean battle. It is hand-to-hand combat. Bloody, dirty, sweaty, bayonet combat. If the strategy of the attack isn't well-enough planned or if there are not enough soldiers to fight the battle, the battle often is lost.

To beat the monster of depression, people need a well-thought-out plan based on a proven strategy.

A strategy that has been tested. And a plan that is simple and clear to follow.

THE SPELLED-OUT PLAN

If I Could Just Snap Out of It, Don't You Think I Would? is a nine-month plan for beating depression and achieving happiness. The centerpiece of this book is a weekly calendar with very specific behavioral (action) and cognitive (thought) activities. Spelled out on each day of the week are activities to follow and the amount of time to be spent on each.

The behavioral activities in this book are based on what is known about the lives of happy people. This is what is known. People who are connected to others are generally happier than those who are not. People who give of themselves feel their lives have meaning. People who have strong support systems are well-equipped to fight their battles. People who take care of their bodies feel good about themselves.

The behavioral activities in this book also reintroduce behaviors that help connect depressed people with others and add meaning and interest to their lives.

The cognitive activities also are based on what is known about happy people. Happy people believe in themselves. They see themselves as well-meaning individuals who make mistakes. Their internal messages are forgiving, unlike the cruel, internal messages of those who are depressed.

The cognitive activities outlined in the calendar help correct the depressed individual's automatic, nasty messages.

Imagine that your mind is a big sponge. From the time you are old enough to understand what is said, your mind soaks up everything it hears and keeps the important messages for later review.

If what you repeatedly hear is, "What a beautiful girl," you learn to feel good about yourself. If what you hear is, "What a useless kid," you learn to hate yourself.

The more positive statements, the more positively you see yourself. The more you've been criticized and demeaned, the more expert you become at berating yourself, sucker-punching yourself with negative thoughts and words.

By the time you are old enough to shave and drain your car oil, the negative messages become your own. Now, when you miss a shot on the basketball court or get a D on a test, you tell yourself what a jerk you are. There is no, "I'll get it next time."

The cognitive activities in this book are based on solid principles:

* Thoughts come before feelings. You don't wake up sad. You feel sad after you awaken and think, "Great, another sucky day."
* What you think matters more than what is. If you think you can do something, you will accomplish your goal. If you think you are incapable, you will fail.
* If someone important to you tells you something enough times, you will believe it. It doesn't matter whether it is true.
* You believe the *shoulds* on which you have been suckled. "People who don't do what they should are bad." And so on.
* Pictures are more powerful than words. Being called "a pig" does more damage than being told to slow down on what you eat.

Like model clay, we humans are shaped and left to dry. Our families and cultures teach us what to believe. Like good students, we learn well. We learn best when statements are simple.

"Thin is good. Fat is bad. Beauty is good. Ugly is bad. Young is good. Old is bad."

The cognitive portion of *If I Could Just Snap Out of It, Don't You Think I Would?* offers you the tools to understand why you think as you do and the ways to change how you think. In so doing, you will change how you feel.

THE BASICS OF THE MOOD-CHANGING PLAN

The basics of the mood-changing plan are both simple and profound. The behaviors and thoughts you are asked to reduce or eliminate are ones that do you disservice. The behaviors and thoughts you are asked to adopt are ones that serve you well.

These are the behaviors you are asked to add or change: watch television for no more than three hours a day (less is better); do not abuse alcohol or drugs; don't sleep more than eight hours a day; choose to eat a healthy diet (a Mediterranean diet or one like it, with an emphasis on fruits, vegetables, seeds, nuts, whole grains, fish, and olive oil is a good choice, as it is reported to help with moods); supplement daily with Omega-3 if you are not getting enough on your own; take a daily vitamin B complex supplement if your doctor says it's O.K.; spend time outside, even in winter, so as to get enough sunshine; go somewhere where there are other people (preferably people you know or with whom you have things in common) twice a week for an hour and while there, take it upon yourself to initiate at least two conversations; choose to volunteer for a cause that matters to you and offer your services to this cause at least once a week for a minimum of two hours; exercise twice a week (at least one of these times with others); add to your exercise by going for two walks a week, alone or with a buddy; engage weekly in an activity you have enjoyed in the past (think picnic on the beach); spend an hour and a half each week learning something you have always wanted to learn; and spend at least a half hour a week somewhere you consider spiritual. While there, make a list of everything that is good in your life. Take the time to appreciate the beauty around you. Thank the universe for your gifts.

The reasons for these activities are simple. People who are depressed have let their bodies, minds, and connections go. They have lost so much control they have forgotten they have power. They have given up hope. Going after life again shows them that they can live. They learn that living is much like getting back on a bicycle. It might take getting used to again, but one never forgets how to ride.

The cognitive activities you are asked to add are as follows: begin every day with a recited promise to conquer your depression; record your daily, automatic thoughts and talkback to these thoughts; decide, specifically, what you want to change about you; once a week, make detailed plans on how you will accomplish these changes; reality-test your negative thoughts; make note of everything that is positive about you and give yourself credit for things well-done; find and work with a mood coach (a mood coach is "a therapist sort-of," a friend or acquaintance who will call you on your self-sabotaging behaviors and applaud you on your hard work) and work with this mood coach once or twice a week for a half hour to an hour a time.

If you agree to follow the mood-changing plan, you will have committed to changing your behaviors and working on your self-perceptions.

If you work the plan steadfastly for at least nine months, your depression will lift. If you work the plan for a year, your depression will become as blurred as that gas station sign three hundred yards back, seen through a scratched rear view mirror. But I will say it straight out. You have to stick with the plan indefinitely. There is no saying, "My work is done. Now I'm free." The reason you will feel better at a year's milestone and two-years' milestone is because you have changed how you think about yourself and what you do. If you forget about the changes you have made, your depression will return.

Depression is a grizzly bear. If you get lazy and drop your depression-fighting activities and exercises like so much food, the grizzly will find you.

THE MOOD-CHANGING CALENDAR

If you are ready to kick your depression to the curb, your next nine months will be spent working with the mood-changing calendar below. While you may not understand now all of what is being asked of you, it will soon become very clear. All of the mood-changing calendar's activities are explained in detail throughout the book. The calendar is very straightforward and easy to follow. Just read, do what you are asked, and let the good times start coming.

Each calendar day requires that you engage in certain activities for specific amounts of time. Activities that are noted to be once or twice a week for one or one-and-a-half hours can be spread out over the week. Certainly, if you work full-time, you may need to spread out the activities. While the "Connect with Others" activity (time spent meeting with others and initiating conversations) is slotted to occur twice a week for an hour a time, it may be more convenient for you to initiate your conversations in bits of time. Who says that conversations can't happen at work—at the water cooler or while you and others wait for the start of a meeting? Even better is the lunch table where you and your coworkers are taking a much needed break. However, if your "Connect with Others" activity takes place in bits of time, make sure that your "bits" add up to the amount of time being asked of you.

Feel free to break up other activities as well. Fifteen minutes here and there still add up to an hour or two. Just be sure to put in the amount of time requested.

Where are you going to find the time to do the activities? From wherever you can!

Remember, this is your life we are talking about. Maybe you'll squeeze in a walk at five in the morning, or you will learn to play the guitar after work, or you'll spend fifteen minutes at noon reflecting on the beauty around you. Depending on your schedule, you may have to do more of the requested activities on the weekends. I know that heaping on more responsibilities on Saturday or Sunday is as appealing as asking you to muck a particularly large horse's stall, but think of it this way. When you shed your depressive skin, everything in life will feel lighter. And brighter.

That being said, you must do your cognitive activities (recording your automatic thoughts, talking-back to your thoughts…) every day for the amount of time asked of you. Cognitive activities address the awful things you say to yourself. You cannot skimp on this work. You have spent years beating yourself up and internalizing just about everything you have ever said. The damage these thoughts have caused you is mind-boggling. The time now has come to challenge your thinking. Only when you change how you talk to and treat yourself, will you change how you see yourself. And only then will your depression begin to lift.

If an activity is hard, don't give up on it. Take a break if you need to, but keep working on it. And give yourself credit. This is hard work.

THE MOOD-CHANGING CALENDAR
REQUIREMENTS FOR EVERY DAY

Limit your sleep to eight hours a day. Do not take naps unless medically necessary. Limit your television watching to a maximum of three hours a day. (Less is better.) Avoid substance abuse. Change to a healthy diet (a Mediterranean diet or one similar, which emphasizes fruits, vegetables, nuts, seeds, fish, and olive oil and limits meat, dairy, and processed foods is a good choice.) Supplement your diet with Omega 3 if you are not getting enough in your diet. Take a Vitamin B complex (but check with your doctor first.) Spend time outside, even in winter. Consider a light box if you do not get enough sunshine or have Seasonal Affective Disorder.

****

MONDAY

(Starred activities are the cognitive activities that must be done every day)

Time-Specific Activities

* 1 : Fight My Depression Pledge-Three Minutes
  2 : Go Out, Connect with People, and Initiate at Least Two Conversations. (If you know people, even casually, who gather anywhere, consider joining them. If you know no one, go somewhere where other people gather. No matter what group you join, you are required to initiate at least two conversations) - One Hour
  3 : Give Myself Three Positive and Honest Statements - Ten Minutes
  4 : Write My Three Positive Statements on Index Cards and Post - Ten Minutes

Activities Ongoing Throughout Day

* 5 : Record My Automatic Thoughts -
      Ongoing throughout Day
* 6 : Record My Talk-Back to My Thoughts -
      Ongoing throughout Day
* 7 : Record My More Realistic Thing to Say to Myself -
      Ongoing throughout Day
* 8 : What Are the Underlying Messages of My Automatic Thoughts? -
      Ongoing throughout Day

* 9 : *What Am I Willing to Do About My Messages? - Ongoing throughout Day*

Total Hours for the Day - Two and a Half Hours

****

TUESDAY

(Starred activities are the cognitive activities that must be done every day.)

Time-Specific Activities

* 1 : *Fight My Depression Pledge-Three Minutes*
  2 : *Engage in an Activity from the B List (These are pleasurable activities.) - One and a Half Hours*
  3 : *Go Somewhere Spiritual - (This can be an organized place of worship or any place that you consider spiritual. Reflect on your life.) - Half Hour*

Activities Ongoing Throughout Day

* 4 : *Record My Automatic Thoughts - Ongoing throughout Day*
* 5 : *Record My Talk-Back to My Thoughts - Ongoing throughout Day*
* 6 : *Record My More Realistic Thing to Say to Myself - Ongoing throughout Day*
* 7 : *What Are the Underlying Messages of My Automatic Thoughts? - Ongoing throughout Day*
* 8 : *What Am I Willing to Do About My Messages? - Ongoing throughout Day*

Total Hours for the Day - Two and a Half to Three Hours

****

WEDNESDAY

(Starred activities are the cognitive activities that must be done every day.)

Time Specific Activities

* 1 : Fight My Depression Pledge-Three Minutes
  2 : Fight My Depression Visualization - Ten Minutes
  3 : Volunteer Somewhere Meaningful to Me - Two Hours
  4 : Go for a Walk, Alone, or with a Friend - Half Hour

Activities Ongoing Throughout Day

* 5 : Record My Automatic Thoughts -
  Ongoing throughout Day
* 6 : Record My Talk-Back to My Thoughts -
  Ongoing throughout Day
* 7 : Record My More Realistic Thing to Say to Myself -
  Ongoing throughout Day
* 8 : What Are the Underlying Messages of My Automatic Thoughts? -
  Ongoing throughout Day
* 9 : What Am I Willing to Do About My Messages?
  Ongoing throughout Day

Total Hours for Day - Three to Three and a Half Hours

****

THURSDAY

(Starred activities are the cognitive activities that must be done every day.)

Time Specific Activities

* 1 : Fight My Depression Pledge-Three Minutes
  2 : Go Out and Connect with People (If you know people, even casually, who gather anywhere, consider joining them. If you know no one, go somewhere where other people gather. No matter what group you join, you are required to initiate at least two conversations.) - One Hour
  3 : Work With My Mood Coach - One Half to One Hour

Activities Ongoing Throughout Day

* 4 : Record My Automatic Thoughts - Ongoing throughout Day
* 5 : Record My Talk-Back to My Thoughts - Ongoing throughout Day
* 6 : Record My More Realistic Thing to Say to Myself - Ongoing throughout Day
* 7 : What Are the Underlying Messages of My Automatic Thoughts? - Ongoing throughout Day
* 8 : What Am I Willing to Do About My Messages? Ongoing throughout Day

Total Hours for Day – Two and a Half to Three Hours

****

FRIDAY

(Starred activities are the cognitive activities that must be done every day.)

Time-Specific Activities

* 1 : Fight My Depression Pledge-Three Minutes
  2 : Exercise With Other People - Thirty Minutes
  3 : Learn Something New - One and a Half Hours

Activities Ongoing Throughout Day

* 4 : Record My Automatic Thoughts -
  Ongoing throughout Day
* 5 : Record My Talk-Back to My Thoughts -
  Ongoing throughout Day
* 6 : Record My More Realistic Thing to Say to Myself -
  Ongoing throughout Day
* 7 : What Are the Underlying Messages of My Automatic Thoughts? -
  Ongoing throughout Day
* 8 : What Am I Willing to Do About My Messages?-
  Ongoing throughout Day

Total Hours for Day - Two and a Half to Three Hours

****

SATURDAY

(Starred activities are the cognitive activities that must be done every day.)

Time-Specific Activities

* 1 : Fight My Depression Pledge-Three Minutes
  2 : Fight My Depression Visualization - Ten Minutes
  3 : How Will I Realize My Goals? *(Make Detailed Weekly Plans)* - Forty-Five Minutes
  4 : Give Thanks Aloud (List the Things for Which I Am Grateful - Ten Minutes
  5 : Go for a Walk, Alone, or with a Friend - Thirty Minutes

Activities Ongoing Throughout Day

* 6 : Record My Automatic Thoughts - Ongoing throughout Day
* 7 : Record My Talk-Back to My Thoughts - Ongoing throughout Day
* 8 : Record My More Realistic Thing to Say to Myself - Ongoing throughout Day
* 9 : What Are the Underlying Messages of My Automatic Thoughts? - Ongoing throughout Day
*10 : What Am I Willing to Do About My Messages? - Ongoing throughout Day

Total Hours for Day - Two and a Half to Three Hours

SUNDAY

Time-Specific Activities

* 1 : Fight My Depression Pledge-Three Minutes
  2 : Exercise (With or Without Others) - Half Hour
  3 : Work with My Mood Coach (If Needed) - One Half to One Hour
  4 : Reward Myself for Work Well-Done - Two Hours

Total Hours for Day - Two and a Half to Three Hours

CHAPTER THREE

WHEN MEDICATION COMES FIRST

MANY PEOPLE WHO ARE VERY depressed and not on medication lack the motivation to do anything—even if that anything is going to make them feel better. While the ideas in this book may make sense to these people, even a lot of sense, there is little they can do to follow the advice. Depression is blocking their paths to well-being.

Chemical imbalances may not right themselves without intervention. Some depressed people need medication before they can do anything else. When people are lifted out of their funks and given the energy to try, they become more able to do the work necessary to get well.

The first step in battling depression is to consider how much your depression stands in your way. How much does it prevent you from living the life you want? If the answer is a lot, then before doing any of the work in this book, you should consider talking to a doctor about whether you would benefit from medication.

Many people balk at the idea of taking psychiatric medication. They believe that medications that change how they think or feel, change their very souls.

This is an interesting subject. Do the workings of our brains change throughout our lives? The answer is yes. Is our chemical makeup the same at birth as it is at age seventeen or forty-seven? The answer is no.

The chemistry of our brain changes as we live our lives. Stress, good or bad, changes this chemistry. Being depressed, chronically in pain, or anxious is stressful. Getting married, landing a new job, or having a child is stressful. Being abused or traumatized is hugely stressful.

When you take your psychiatric medication, you are helping your brain reduce the effects of stress and return to the general area of a "baseline you."

We don't question the need to take medication for high blood pressure. Yet, the brain is as much an organ of the body as the heart. What we refer to as a good mind is not more or less than an optimally functioning brain. Do what you need to do to ensure that your brain functions optimally.

That being said, not everyone needs medication. Some people can do the work without it.

So what's the litmus test? How do you know if you need medication?

Start by questioning the severity of your depression. Does a crushing sadness prevent you from getting up in the morning? Does hopelessness keep you sleeping much of the day or prevent you from sleeping at night? Has a recurrent irritability made you snap at most everyone? Have you lost your appetite for foods you used to love or have you taken to eating much more than usual? Does a sense of despair keep you crying much of the time? Are you avoiding the people with whom you used to spend all your time? Have you lost interest in the things about which you used to be passionate? Does life feel like a burden, like a series of endless tasks you have to accomplish?

If the answer to one or more of these questions is yes, if these symptoms have lasted for more than two weeks and you can't shake them, you should see a doctor and consider medication.

There are many medications used to treat depression. The majority of them are antidepressants known as SSRIs—Selective Serotonin Reuptake Inhibitors. Serotonin is a chemical in the brain that is associated with mood. A normal level of serotonin promotes feelings of well-being. When there is not enough serotonin available, our moods can suffer. SSRIs work by maintaining an ample supply of available serotonin in the brain. Some commonly known SSRIs are Prozac, Paxil, Zoloft, and Celexa.

WHEN SAFETY COMES FIRST

Sometimes, those with severe depression lose the ability to see through their pain. Like those whose lives are destroyed by rogue waves, they lose so much. Hopes and dreams are ripped away and shattered, left to lie among the rubble. Connection and involvement are sucked out to sea. Even the sunshine seems gone. In all the bleakness and muck, death seems preferable. They cannot see that tomorrow or the next day, the sun again will shine, and an army of volunteers will arrive to help them salvage their lives.

This book is intended for people who are depressed. However, for those who have been thinking about suicide and have decided to act, the material in this book must wait. Your safety is what matters.

If you believe that you cannot protect yourself, you need to take action immediately. Call 911. Do so even before calling your family. Police and fire fighters will respond and take you to the hospital. Do not be embarrassed. Nobody is going to make fun of you. To the contrary, people will admire you for asking for help.

If you find yourself preoccupied with thoughts of suicide, even if you have no plan, you also must take action. Put this book aside for now and call a family member or close friend in whom you can confide. Call your therapist. If the thoughts persist and you fear you may act on them, go to your local emergency room. Explain to the triage staff that you are having suicidal thoughts. A doctor and a psychiatric screener will meet with you. Talking with them will make you feel better and will help you figure out your options. They may suggest that you find a therapist and a psychiatrist or go into a partial hospitalization program (an intensive outpatient day program lasting from a few days to two weeks). If you are unsure about your safety, they will help you to be hospitalized.

Once you have gotten help and are no longer suicidal, start working the steps in this book. And use what you have learned from your experience to help others. Having moved beyond your despair, you are in a great position to be a beacon of hope to others.

CHOOSING A DOCTOR

If you think you could benefit from medication, it is essential that you see a doctor.

My advice: choose your doctor wisely.

While all medical doctors can prescribe psychiatric medication, only psychiatrists have the specific training in treating psychiatric disorders.

Consider your situation. Is your depression mild and annoying or are you so depressed that you can't get out of bed?

If your situation is mild, perhaps you can begin treatment by talking to your primary care doctor.

If your situation is complicated, find the best psychiatrist you can.

To find such a doctor, you need to do your research. Check out hospitals with well-known psychiatric departments. Read the doctor's biography on line. Look for psychiatrists who specialize in mood disorders. See which doctors are leading workshops, giving talks, and/or conductiong research in the field.

Ask people you respect for recommendations. Ask your primary care doctor for a suggestion.

Do not insist that your psychiatrist be within a thirty minute drive. Once you get on the medication that works, you may need only to see your psychiatrist once every two or three months.

Find a psychiatrist who will listen to you, but don't confuse the ability to listen with a pleasant personality.

While a good bedside manner is nice, it is not essential. One of the best psychiatrists I know has a very odd presentation. He hasn't the slightest idea when I am telling a joke.

He pauses too long between thoughts. He is too serious. He is brilliant.

CHARTING YOUR MOODS

Before you see your doctor, write down everything you can think of about your moods. Be specific. What is your sadness like? Do you spend the day in bed? Do you sleep too much or have trouble sleeping? Record the number of hours you sleep per night. Has your appetite increased or decreased? Do you cry a lot? Have you lost interest in things you used to enjoy? Do you have trouble concentrating? Do you isolate? Are you thinking about suicide? Do you have a plan? Have you done anything to hurt yourself? Do you feel hopeless?

Keep a mood chart so as to have a visual indicator of your moods. Copy the one below or make your own. The mood chart will help your doctor determine the best medication for you. After you start your medication, it will help determine how well the medication is working and will help your psychiatrist make changes.

Take an active role in your medication treatment. Only you know how you feel on your medication. Write down any side effects you experience. Speak up. You have fifteen to thirty minutes for an appointment. Make sure your concerns get heard. Too often, people are afraid to talk to their psychiatrists. They feel their concerns are not valid or that they are taking up too much time. Your psychiatrist is there for you. If he/she won't listen to you, find another psychiatrist.

DAILY MOOD CHART

DATE _____

TOOK MEDICATION TODAY   Y   N

HOURS OF SLEEP LAST NIGHT   _____

RATING SCALE   0 = NONE   10 = MOST

DEPRESSION	IRRITABILITY/ANGER	ENERGY
7a.m. _____ /	_____ /	_____
11a.m. _____ /	_____ /	_____
3p.m _____ /	_____ /	_____
7p.m. _____ /	_____ /	_____
11p.m. _____ /	_____ /	_____

APPETITE	SLEEP	SUICIDALITY
7a.m. _____ /	_____ /	_____
11a.m. _____ /	_____ /	_____
3p.m _____ /	_____ /	_____
7p.m. _____ /	_____ /	_____
11p.m. _____ /	_____ /	_____

NOTES/REFLECTIONS

_____
_____
_____
_____

TAKING YOUR MEDICATION

Most of us are accustomed to taking medication when we feel lousy. If we have a headache, we take aspirin. If we have a really bad headache, we take Extra Strength Excedrin or something similar. These medications take about ten minutes to work. We only take these medications when we need them. Continuing to take headache medication when we no longer have a headache makes no sense.

Most psychiatric medications work differently from the drugs you buy over the counter. They build up in the blood stream. That's why it often takes six to eight weeks to feel their full effect. Psychiatric medication needs to be taken every day and as many times a day as prescribed. If you take several medications, you may find it helpful to use a pill box with the days of the week labeled and slots for a.m. and p.m. medication.

It is typical for those who have never taken medications to feel uncomfortable with the thought of taking them. To them, medication is their scarlet letter, their proof that something is wrong. But antidepressant medications are some of the most widely prescribed medications in America. And it is strong people who address their frailties and do something about them.

CHAPTER FOUR

FACING YOUR ANGER

It's time to face your anger. Head on.

Life isn't fair. You hate being depressed. Other people don't have to fight like you do. Why are you seeing your psychiatrist when other guys are out playing poker or hitting on girls? You were supposed to be born with normal genes. Life is supposed to be fun. You don't know what fun is. You're mad. Fighting mad. Smash somebody mad.

O.K. It's good to get angry. In fact, getting angry, really angry, is the first step in beating your depression. So give your anger all you've got. Put your anger in a corner and square off with it. Take off your boxing gloves. This is time to get bloody. But direct your anger appropriately. It's nobody's fault. Even if you inherited your depression from your father, don't blame him. He didn't want it either.

Besides, no one said life is fair.

"Wait a minute," you say. "I'm a good guy. I'm supposed to get some good stuff out of life. Life's supposed to be fair."

O.K., tell that to the babies dying of starvation. Tell it to the army vet who served his country and came home with no legs.

Being born doesn't guarantee that you're going to get a fair shake.

THE PROBLEM WITH ANGER

The problem with anger is that you have to figure out what you're going to do with it. Feeling sorry for yourself is one thing, blaming the world is another. Some people are so angry, feeling their lot in life so unfair, they hate the world. They feed on their hate. They don't blame themselves; they blame everyone else. You know these people. You've read about them. They beat their wives. Their kids. They spend their money on alcohol and drugs.

Other people stuff their feelings. Maybe they don't take their anger out on others, but they are so stuck, they don't help themselves. They give into their depression. They find excuses. "It's all too hard," they say. "I'd fight it if I could. I've tried. But nothing works. The meds are lousy. The therapist doesn't get it. The doctor's a jerk. What am I supposed to do?"

Still other people take their intense feelings out on themselves. They hate being depressed. They feel like cowards. They say things like, "I'm taking up space. Sucking up air." They stockpile razors. They cut themselves. They think about suicide.

All of these reactions are understandable. People who are depressed didn't get to pick their battles.

But no one else does either.

Some people's fights are bigger than others'. Children's cancer wards are full. Life takes bravery and courage. Life's about putting your butt on the chair and doing the work. People often die from cancer without chemotherapy. People who are horribly injured in automobile accidents only learn to walk and talk again by suffering through months and years of rehabilitation.

What you do with your depression is up to you. How hard you fight is your choice. But think about this. You only get one shot at this life.

Try this exercise. Imagine you are on your death bed. Your breathing is labored. You only have a few minutes left in this world. Reflect on your life. What was good? What wasn't? Did you give it all you had? Would you change anything if you could get more time to do so? Then remember, it's just an exercise. You've been given a gift. You have time to change things. What will you change?

A person once said, "The best defense against death is a life well-lived."

How well are you going to live yours?

ANGER AND RESISTANCE GO TOGETHER

"O.K.," you say. "I'm tired of the pity pot. But this thing, this depression, is bigger than I am. It's a huge, terrifying grizzly that stalks me every time I go for a walk in the woods. I want it to go away. But I don't know how. I don't even know where to begin."

You begin by realizing that your anger over your depression and your sense of being unfairly targeted by the universe has cost you dearly. You accept that as much as you want to be rid of your depression, you haven't done what it takes to make it go away. You've been resistant to fighting your depression.

"Wait a minute," you say. "I want my depression to go away. I don't have resistance."

Yes, I know. The resistance is to the hard, sometimes grueling, and time-consuming work that's necessary.

Your next step is to decide that you will be defeated by your depression no longer. You will do whatever it takes to get better. You will address your resistance directly.

"How do I do this?" you ask.

You start by creating a pledge that you will say to yourself every single day when you awaken. As they do in AA, you will take on your fight against depression and against your resistance to fighting your depression one day at a time.

Feel free to write your own Depression-Fighting pledge. This is the one I share with my clients.

"*I hate the fact that I have depression and it makes me angry that I have to fight a battle that so many other people don't have to fight. But my depression has already robbed me of so much. I'm tired of being sad. I want to live. I want to savor the beauty of life, to challenge myself and to live fully and richly. This is the only life I have in this world and I want to live it. I will fight my depression. I will fight it hard. I will fight it today. And every day. And I will win.*"

If you want to write your own "I Will Fight My Depression" pledge, you can do so here.

_____
_____
_____
_____
_____
_____
_____
_____
_____
_____
_____
_____
_____
_____

Now that you have your depression-fighting pledge in place, I am going to teach you an exercise that you can use along with your pledge. You don't have to do this exercise every day, but you should follow your pledge with it at least twice a week.

DEPRESSION-FIGHTING EXERCISE

Along with your pledge, the Depression-Fighting exercise will aid you in your fight against sadness. This exercise employs deep breathing, which is an excellent relaxation technique, and visualization, a technique which allows you to see as fully executed the goals you wish to accomplish.

Go into an empty room where you will not be disturbed. Turn off all electronic devices. Sit in a comfortable chair. Close your eyes and relax. With your mouth closed, take a very deep breath through your nose. Fill your lungs completely with the air. When you feel that you cannot possibly take in any more air, slowly start counting to three. Count like you did when you were a kid: One Mississippi, two Mississippi, three Mississippi. Then, make a tight circle with your lips and blow out very slowly. Control your air flow. You should feel your shoulders relax. After you release all the air from your lungs, make the circle with your lips again and blow out more air. Do this slowly. Now you should feel the muscles in your stomach relax. Repeat this exercise three times.

Now you are going to do the visualization part of the exercise. In this part, you will imagine yourself as a soldier, fighting your enemy: your depression.

With your eyes closed, visualize yourself on a hilly battleground. See yourself as strong and tall and holding a rifle with one hand. See your other hand resting on a cannon. Look across the field and see many soldiers. They are your opposers, your enemies. Zoom in on the different soldiers. See the fat one; see the tall and skinny one. Imagine each as representing a different part of your depression. As you look from soldier to soldier, identify the role that each plays in your depression. Perhaps the first soldier is the part of your depression that makes you sleep so much. Perhaps the next soldier is the part that makes you so irritable or makes you lose interest in the things you used to love.

Now, staring down the soldiers, lift your rifle and take aim. After, go to your cannon and shoot. Take down your enemies. End victorious.

When you finish your visualization, repeat your "I Will Fight My Depression" pledge.

EXPRESS YOUR ANGER EFFCTIVELY

People who stuff their anger often get depressed.

One of the women with whom I work is constantly criticized by her brother. Unfortunately for her, they live together. If this woman buys oatmeal, her brother asks why she didn't buy sweetened cereal. If she buys cereal, he asks her why she's buying the fattening stuff. If she pays their rent on time, he asks her why she didn't pay another bill first. If she pays another bill first, he questions why she is late on the rent.

She never responds to his criticisms. She stuffs her feelings. She's often depressed.

Learning to express your anger is important. It says to you, and to anyone who is listening, that your feelings matter.

Anger serves an important function. It is our alarm system, alerting us to problems. It tells us when things are not right, when we are being exploited, manipulated, deceived, or betrayed. It tells us that things need to be fixed.

Many people are afraid to express their anger. They believe that if they get angry with casual acquaintances, these people won't like them. They believe if they get angry with the people they love, these people will leave them.

The trick is in how you express your anger. And the basic rules are these: Criticize the behavior, not the person. Use "I" statements. Tell the person how his behavior makes you feel. And suggest a way that all parties can win.

If your partner leaves his stuff everywhere, it is better to tell him that messes make you crazy than to tell him that he is a slob.

"I get nuts when you leave things a mess."

Suggest a win-win solution.

"If you can just pick up after yourself, I'll stop bugging you. Then we'll both win."

Getting your frustration, your anger, out will do a lot to lift your depression. Do it appropriately and you will be saying to yourself and the world, "I matter."

DEAL WITH YOUR GUILT AND SAY YOU ARE SORRY

Many depressed people hate themselves. Often it is because of guilt. One of my clients says he had the most terrific beginnings and yet has accomplished nothing other than becoming an awesome alcoholic. He feels horribly guilty. Another client's self-esteem plummeted after he left his high school girlfriend when she was pregnant with their child. A third client's guilt tortures him because he holds himself responsible for his uncle's death, although everyone in his family tells him it was an accident that could not have been avoided. Another client's guilt does a number on her every February, before and after the fourteenth of the month, the anniversary of the day she hit a boy while driving.

Guilt is destructive. You need to deal with it.

What do you do? Look your guilt squarely in the eyes. Address yourself honestly. Ask yourself what happened. Take responsibility for what you did. Judge yourself fairly. Don't give yourself unnecessary slack or judge yourself against superhuman standards. Mourn the fact that you can't change the past. Apologize to the universe. Apologize to the people you hurt. If appropriate, ask them for forgiveness. If not, offer an apology from the soul and don't expect anything in return. Accept that you can't change what happened.

What else can you do? Try reaching out. Help people learn from your mistakes. If your actions were the result of drugs or alcohol, help other people maintain sobriety. If your actions were the result of uncontrolled anger, help others learn to control their rage.

Ultimately, what is done is done. From here on, you will do the absolute best that you can.

That needs to be enough.

LETTING GO

Letting go of anger is not forgetting. It's deciding to move on. It's realizing that your anger is destroying you.

Anger eats you up, keeps you stuck, and stops you from growing. If you can let go of your anger, do so. If you need help to let go, get it. If letting go is simply impossible, if the event was just too big, too horrible, then turn your anger into something positive. Help others avoid what hurt you so badly. Turn your pain into a force for change.

SHARE YOUR SCARS

O.K. Maybe your father, mother, uncle, or caretaker didn't deserve any of your love. Maybe the universe should have arranged for any one of them to be pecked to death by a nasty old bird at one of those cockfights they loved so much more than you. Maybe that would have been payback for the years of abuse and humiliation you suffered at their hands. Yes indeed, maybe, because after all, your unwillingness to talk to them hasn't done the trick. It hasn't healed your wounds. Nope, the wounds are still seeping. So what's a person like you, damaged so deeply, to do?

Stop paying the price for another's cruelty. Stop being a victim. The only one you are hurting is yourself. Take back control. Realize that while you might be scarred, you are not damaged. Give your scars the respect they deserve. They are proof of your endurance. If your scars are visible, touch them. Stroke them. Their very existence cost you so much. If your scars are internal, pick a place on your arms or legs and make it your scar spot. With washable magic marker, capture the essence of your scar with a design or a picture. Perhaps you will draw a dragon. It will be your way of telling cruel adversaries to beware: your breath has turned to fire. Perhaps your picture will be that of a butterfly, your way of saying that from here on in, you will fly where you choose and come to rest only where sweetness beckons.

When you share your scars, you hide them no more. And without secrets to keep, life is much lighter.

WRITE YOUR EPITAPH

I don't want to be buried. But just in case my children haven't listened the fifty-plus times I have told them that I wish to be cremated, I have given thought to my epitaph. I think I would like it to read: "She loved her children, she loved to think, she tried to make a difference in the world." Why these words and not other words? Simply, because this is what matters to me.

I have come to see that an epitaph is a way of capturing the essence of a life. It's an opportunity to boil away all that is inconsequential and leave only the crucial sweet kernels of truth and importance.

I also have come to realize that thinking about our epitaphs is a way for us to contemplate what we want our lives to mean. What legacy do you want to leave to the world? Start by considering what matters most to you. Is it kindness to others? Is it giving of the self? Is it intellectual or athletic prowess? Is it following your creative muse? Is it thinking so far outside the box that you change how we humans see ourselves? Is it sitting in or marching on for peace? Is it generosity?

Write your epitaph, long before you need it. Then live by it.

TAKE RESPONSIBILITY

No matter what you have lived through, no matter how terrible, you need to arrive at a place where you say, "It's my life, and from here on in, I take full responsibility for it." If the damage done to you is thick and deep like brownish, red clay, seek help and work through it. If the damage has hardened into sandstone, take your chisel out and crack away at what you can.

If no one has ever loved you, learn to love yourself.

If you are lonely, reach out to someone lonelier. Free a dog from a shelter and make her yours. Spend Sundays at a nursing home. Ladle soup at a soup kitchen. Become a better friend.

Stop focusing on those who have hurt you. You've given them enough. Don't let them take your whole life. What you make of your life from here on in is up to you. Make it count.

"How?" you say.

Take stock of your abilities. Decide what you want from life. Realize that anything worth getting takes work. Acknowledge that getting there will be difficult. Work on self-discipline. And tell yourself you owe this… to you.

CHAPTER FIVE

ONE, TWO, THREE AND THE DAMAGE IS DONE or THOUGHTS CAN DO YOU IN

ARE THE THOUGHTS OF DEPRESSED people really that bad?

The answer is simple. Yes.

Depressed people find it nearly impossible to see themselves in a positive light. But ask what is wrong with them and the answers flow freely. This is particularly true when it comes to their internal thoughts, referred to throughout this book and in most of cognitive literature as "automatic thoughts." Automatic thoughts are our twenty-four/seven commentary on everything we do, say, or feel. They are called automatic thoughts because they come to us unbeckoned, uncensored, and almost always, unwelcome. In depressed individuals, these thoughts are harsh, nasty, and lopsided. They are words and phrases imprinted in youth—the product of others' unrealistic expectations, criticism, or abuse. They are the stuff of our internal tapes, the voices of our internal critics.

"You're a jerk."
"You're a loser."
"You're a fat pig."

All day long, depressed people rip themselves up, tear themselves apart, and leave organ parts out to dry in the sun.

If you believe your false, lopsidedly negative commentary, you cannot overcome your depression.

To overcome depression, you must challenge your automatic thoughts.

THE FIVE-STEP PROCESS

In an effort to get my clients to see the critical nature of their automatic thoughts, I ask them to capture these thoughts on paper. To do this, I ask them to write down the thoughts when they think them. Exactly as they think them.

"I'm such a huge asshole. Do you hear me? Such a huge asshole."

If this is your thought, this is what goes on paper. Word for word. Capturing your thought, exactly as you hear it, is step number one of the five-step process.

Recording these thoughts is much too important a task to do on scraps of paper. Instead, buy a notebook and carry it everywhere. When thoughts come to you, record them. The ability to review these thoughts is essential for your process of change.

Step number two is learning to "talk back" to your thoughts. Talking back requires that you throw your judgmental self, your internalized self-critic, to the curb and become a more neutral commentator. It also requires that you dig for answers in the muck of your automatic thoughts. Why are you saying what you are? Is this what you believe or what you think others believe? Are you simply repeating what you have been told in the past? Are you being too hard on yourself? Would twenty objective people agree with your assessment?

Look at your language and debunk it. Why are you comparing yourself to a whale? You don't weigh a ton or live in the sea.

Step three requires that you rewrite your automatic thoughts in a more neutral fashion.

If today you awakened and called yourself a "cockroach" because you stole from your brother last night; if yesterday a friend called herself a "troll" because she finds her appearance so unappealing; if a buddy walked into a street calling, "Hey somebody, run me over. Get rid of one more worthless drunk," all three of you need to neutralize your statements.

Throwing these sort of bone-crushing punches does little except assure that nothing will change. Change occurs in an environment of acceptance. Neutralizing your statements will facilitate change.

If you stole from your brother, you will reap more benefit from a statement such as, "I am very disappointed in myself because I stole from my brother." Calling yourself a cockroach shrouds you in drama and gives you a place to hide. Saying you are disappointed in yourself puts you out there for all to see. The same is true for the others who have called themselves names. The alcoholic will reap more by saying, "I dislike myself for drinking every day and for being unwilling to stop." Calling himself "one more worthless drunk" is flamboyant and allows him to avoid confronting himself. It does not hold him accountable.

Step number four is to identify the underlying messages of your automatic thoughts. Using the first example above, your message might be, "I don't want to be a thief. I don't want to betray those I love." In the case of the alcoholic, it might be, "I don't like what I am doing. I don't want to drink anymore."

It's the tough stuff that follows in step number five. You must pit your determination against your resistance and see which wins. It's helpful that you have realized something important about yourself, but the fifty-dollar question is this: What are you willing to do about what you have realized? How hard are you willing to work? O.K., so you don't like that you stole from your brother. But are you angry enough at yourself to apologize, accept responsibility, and change? Are you willing to set a goal? What goal will you set?

In a few pages, we will get to the culminating step—laying out the concrete plan for achieving your goal. In this final step, specificity matters. It is in here that you will detail exactly what you will do to make your goal a reality. But I am getting ahead of myself.

To do the work necessary for steps one through five, you need a form suited for working through this process. The form that I use with my clients is the one below. You may want to consider making many copies of this.

Automatic thoughts should be worked on one at a time. It may not be feasible to work on all your thoughts, so be selective. Choose those that do you the most damage.

AUTOMATIC THOUGHT FORM

AUTOMATIC THOUGHT

_____
_____
_____
_____
_____
_____
_____

TALK-BACK TO MY THOUGHT

_____
_____
_____
_____
_____
_____
_____

A MORE REALISTIC THING TO SAY TO MYSELF

_____
_____
_____

WHAT MESSAGE AM I GIVING MYSELF?

_____
_____
_____
_____
_____
_____
_____
_____

WHAT AM I WILLING TO DO ABOUT MY MESSAGE?

_____
_____
_____
_____
_____
_____
_____
_____

O.K. Enough for the talk. Let's get down to work.

What follows are the automatic thoughts of some of my clients, all of whom have given permission for a likeness-monologue to be used. A likeness-monologue is a monologue that has the same flavor and asks the same general questions as the client's monologue. However, in order to protect my clients' confidentiality, I have changed all the names, details, and specifics. But the essence of each monologue remains true. See for yourself what damage automatic thoughts can do.

Maria was a client. When she catalogued an internal monologue similar to the one that follows, she was thirty-five years old and, by her account, thirty-five pounds overweight.

"I'm fat. I look like a pig. Here I am, Porky, going out on the town. All ready and set to be roasted. My body alone could feed all of downtown Boston. Jeez, I'm disgusting. Thoughts of going to Aruba are a joke. I can't fly on a plane. I can't fit into a seat. 'Here she comes, ladies and gentlemen, Porky. Give her two seats, maybe three. What the hell, she's got fat to spare.' I'll never get a date. No one would want to be seen with me. No wonder I'm single. My fat and I will die together. The perfect greasy pair. I hate myself."

"A ridiculous example," you say. "People don't think like that."
They do.
"A farfetched example," you say. "People don't get that carried away with their thoughts."
They do.
These kinds of internal monologues are commonplace, going on in the heads of tens of thousands of people all day long.
Let's see how Maria used the five-step process to deal with her thoughts. See how she targets her thoughts one at a time and only those thoughts she considers most damaging.

Automatic Thought (Maria's first)
"I'm fat."
Talk-Back to My Thought
"How fat is fat? Am I three hundred pounds overweight? Am I five hundred pounds overweight? No, I am not."

A More Realistic Thing to Say to Myself
"I'm thirty-five pounds overweight. I don't like this, but at least I'm not a hundred pounds overweight. Maybe I can do something about it."

What Message Am I Giving Myself?
"I hate the fact that I am overweight."

What Am I Willing to Do About My Message?
"I'm going to come up with a way to start losing some weight. Maybe I'll start by cutting my food in half."

Here's Maria's next automatic thought and her talk-back.

Automatic Thought (her second)
"I look like a pig."

Talk-back to My Thought
"Well, that's ridiculous. Pigs have four legs. I have two. And pigs have a snout. I have a nose. And pigs are short. I'm not. Pigs live in the mud. I avoid the mud at all costs."

A More Realistic Thing to Say to Myself
"I am overweight, but I am not an animal who lives in the mud. I have speech and feelings. In fact, I am very much a human."

What Message Am I Giving Myself?
"Being overweight upsets me so much that I don't even feel human."

What Am I Willing to Do About My Message?
"I will come up with a way to lose weight."

And so on with her automatic thoughts.

Maria also makes numerous assumptions. Thus, in her talk-back, she needs to address these as well. For those who use assumptions, the same automatic thought form can be used.

Automatic Assumption (Maria's first)
"I'm so fat I can't travel because I can't fit into an airline seat."

Talk-Back to My Assumption
"Airlines wouldn't be so stupid as to make their seats so small that people of all sizes can't fit in them. Lots of people are overweight and airlines want business. They are not going to size their seats for skinny people only. Besides, thirty-five pounds is not that much overweight and it won't prevent me from fitting into a seat."

A More Realistic Thing to Say to Myself
"I may have to squeeze into the airline seat, but lots of other people have to do this because there are a lot of people who are overweight. I may feel uncomfortable if people are watching me, but the truth is that most people will be too busy with their own stuff to watch me. But I definitely don't like the fact that I am overweight."

What Message Am I Giving Myself?
"I don't like being overweight."

What Am I Willing to Do About My Message?
"I'm going to lose weight."

Let's look at Maria's next assumption.

Automatic Assumption (her second)
"I'll never get a date."

Talk-Back to My Assumption
"How in the world would I know that? Lots of people get dates. Men are attracted to all sorts of women. Some men like women with fuller figures. Besides, my face is cute. And how can I possibly say I'll never get a date? Do I know what's going to happen to me for the rest of my life?"

A More Realistic Thing to Say to Myself
"Some men may be attracted to me, particularly men who like women with full figures."

What Message Am I Giving Myself?
"I think I'm too fat and I believe I'll have more luck dating if I lose weight."

What Am I Willing to Do About My Message?
"I'm going to lose weight."

Here is another example.

Jim is a thirty-seven-year-old divorced man who lives outside of Boston and works for a factory, a job he has had for eighteen years. It was early in our therapy that he wrote an internal monologue similar to this.

"Another shitty day in paradise. I hate my job. My job sucks. What the hell am I getting up for? The boss is a jerk. The other guys are assholes. Why even bother? Look at the snow. Are they ever going to plow this road? Probably not. After all, it's just us up here—a bunch of stupid losers working for the factories. Bet they plowed the rich suckers' roads. Bet the country club road is plowed. Got to get it right for those country club boys. I hate those rich mothers. Hey, I wouldn't mind taking that chick out. She wouldn't go though. She's probably stuck up. Bet her daddy pays for everything. Bet her sheets are satin. Stupid chick."

Let's look at the work that Jim did with these thoughts.

Automatic Thought (Jim's first)
"I hate my job."

Talk-Back to My Thought
"If I hated my job so much, I wouldn't have worked there for eighteen years."

A More Realistic Thing to Say to Myself
"I don't always hate my job. Some days I do, but some days I like it. Plus, they treat me O.K."

What Message Am I Giving Myself?
"I'm trying to figure out whether I should stay at this job. I am realizing that eight hours a day is too much of my time to be unhappy, if that is what I am."

What Am I Willing to Do About My Message?
"I'm going to make a list of pros and cons about my job. I'm going to decide whether I should stay there or look for new work."

Let's look at another of Jim's automatic thoughts.

Automatic Thought (his second)
"I'm a stupid loser working for a factory."
Talk-Back to My Thought
"I'm not stupid. In fact, I've always thought I was pretty smart. And I'm not a loser. What's a loser anyway? Someone who loses."
A More Realistic Thing to Say to Myself
"What have I lost? My marriage, yes. But that might be for the best. I have a job. A lot of guys don't have work."
What Message Am I Giving Myself?
"It seems I don't feel good about the work I do."
What Am I Willing to Do About My Message?
"I need to decide if factory work is what I want to do. Does my work make me feel good enough about myself?"

And yet another example.

Nikki is eighteen years old. She attends a local university. Most people find her strikingly beautiful. She's had a boyfriend for two-plus years. They love each other and have always been faithful. She worries that he will be unfaithful. She worries that she isn't attractive enough. She wishes she had blond hair. She thinks she is too tall. She worries that she's not a good person because she gets angry too often, particularly at her boyfriend.

Here's an internal dialogue similar to the one she wrote.

"Where the hell is Jason? He was supposed to be here already. Maybe he doesn't want to come over. Maybe he doesn't love me. He's probably sick of me. He's probably out looking for someone else. He'll probably find someone who's nicer to him than I am. Someone prettier. A blond. Someone who's a normal size, not a giraffe like me. Why would he want to be with me anyway? I'm a bitch. Where the hell is he? He's late. I'm going to break up with him."

Let's look at how Nikki talked back to her thoughts.

AUTOMATIC THOUGHT (Nikki's first)
"Jason doesn't want to come over. He's blowing me off."

Talk-Back to My Thought
"Just because Jason is twenty minutes late, doesn't mean he's not coming. He probably got hung up doing something or maybe baseball practice ended late."

A More Realistic Thing to Say to Myself
"I worry too much and jump to conclusions when Jason is late or has a change of plans. I shouldn't worry so much."

What Message Am I Giving Myself?
"I'm afraid that Jason will get sick of me because I get bitchy so much and one day he may just stop coming over."

What Am I Willing to Do About My Message?
"I'm going to start identifying the triggers for my anger and start working on controlling my anger."

Here is another of Nikki's automatic thoughts.

AUTOMATIC THOUGHT (Nikki's second)
"Jason doesn't love me."

Talk-Back to My Thought
"Just because he is twenty minutes late doesn't mean he doesn't love me. Didn't he tell me he loved me yesterday? And the day before? Why would I think that he would feel differently today?"

A More Realistic Thing to Say to Myself
"Jason loves me. I just doubt this when I get upset."

What Message Am I Giving Myself?
"I'm insecure that Jason will stop loving me because I get mad so much. I worry that Jason will find someone who is nicer than me and fall in love with her."

What Am I Willing to Do About my Message?
"I'm going to figure out what makes me angry and get better at controlling it."

CHAPTER SIX

REACHING YOUR GOALS

YOU HAVE BEEN STUCK IN the thick, bubbling quicksand of your automatic thoughts and have had the time to study them. Now you are aware of where your thoughts come from and which are most damaging to you. You have neutralized your statements and now understand the underlying messages of your thoughts. This has allowed you to set goals.

Perhaps your goal is to quit smoking or drinking, go back to school, start dating, or make amends with your family. The goal feels right.

But how do you go from giving something a lot of thought to changing your behavior?

This is where people get stuck. Changing that which you have done for a very long time is difficult. It takes determination, organization, self-discipline, and lots of hard work. It takes doing things that don't always feel good. It takes doing things that cause lots of anxiety.

But you can do it.

This is how.

You start by making a list of questions to which you give honest answers. You then create a plan and determine that you will work your plan whether you want to or not. Feeling like doing it has nothing to do with "doing it."

Suppose you have called yourself a "weak sister" because you hate the fact that you smoke. Smoking makes you feel like you have no will of your own, that you are a slave to your nicotine habit. You have decided you want to quit.

That's great. It's a terrific goal. But how do you get there?

Start with your questions. And give each an honest answer.

How determined are you to quit? Rate your determination.

Why do you smoke? Be honest. Do cigarettes feel like friends? Would giving them up feel as if you're giving up a best high school buddy? Does smoking make you look cool? Did you start smoking at a time when it was believed to be hip and now you can't stop? Are cigarettes your way of coping with anxiety? Have you smoked for so long you can't imagine living without cigarettes?

Why do you want to quit? Here, too, you have to be honest. Do you feel like you are a slave to your cigarettes? Do you hate smelling like you've just come from a sweaty, backroom, whiskey-slugging poker game? Are you sick of the brownish-yellow stains on your teeth? Are you tired of the gray, ghost-like pallor of your face? Are you afraid of getting lung cancer? Do you pant just going up the stairs? Did you promise your kids?

Next, get to the part that matters most.

How will you quit? Will you do it cold-turkey? This plan sounds good, but a lot of people don't make it this way. Will you cut your nicotine down every few days, ending with a cigarette that tastes more like air than thin paper stuffed with tar and nicotine? Will you join a program? Will you do hypnosis? Will you make behavioral changes? If so, what behaviors will you change? Will you put off smoking a cigarette for fifteen minutes after every meal? Will you hold your cigarette in a different hand? Will you smoke from the other side of your mouth?

Decide when you will quit. Do you want to choose a quitting date that is special?

Be very specific with your answers. And write everything down. The written word is more powerful than the spoken.

Tell everyone you know about your decision to quit and the date.

And now another example.

Suppose it's been years since you've had a date and you have decided that the time has come to get out there. How do you begin?

Again, you start with questions. And you answer them honestly.

Are you looking to find a date or are you looking to get married?

What qualities matter to you in a date/partner? Which of these are so important that you have to have them?

What are your deal-breakers?

What are the obstacles that might prevent you from meeting the sort of person for whom you are looking?

Are you willing to do something about your obstacles? In other words, are you willing to change you?

How will you find this person? Are you going to ask your friends to introduce you to all the single people they know? Will you use dating sites? Will you run a personal ad? Will you ask your mother to be on the lookout?

And so it goes.

LAY OUT YOUR PLAN BY THE DAY AND THE HOUR

You have your plan in mind. Now you need to put it on paper. You need to lay out your daily plans in detail.

Feel free to use the "Realizing My Goal–Weekly Plan" form (below) for your specifics.

Make daily and very specific assignments for yourself. Specify the amount of time you will spend on each assignment. Two and a half to three hours a day is good. Less than that and you may feel like you are not working hard enough. More than that and you may burn yourself out.

Build in daily rewards for work done. Yes, you are committed to your goal, but doing what you must is still hard work. Rewards don't have to cost much: a walk on the beach, a video game, a brownie, an episode of your favorite television show.

Build in a long-range reward too. One that you will give yourself when you've accomplished your goal. Perhaps, after years of thinking about quitting smoking, you have been smoke-free for nine months. Or perhaps, after years of thinking about dating, you've joined three dating sites and have had five dates.

The long-term reward you choose should be substantial: a day trip, a weekend trip, that stunning dress, those golf clubs. You've worked very hard to reach your goal. To make these kinds of rewards happen, set aside some money every week. While money is tight for most of us, most people have a dollar or two or five to set aside weekly. If necessary to make it happen, give up something. Forgo your daily Dunkin' Donuts coffee or donut. If you set aside five dollars a week for a year, you will have two hundred and sixty dollars at the end of the year. That's a sweet night away.

THE CONCRETE PLAN IN ACTION

The key to concrete planning is specificity. Detail everything.

Let's look at how you might create a concrete plan for dating. For the purposes of this example, I am assuming you have decided to use dating sites as a way to meet people.

DATING - A SPECIFIC PLAN

Day 1 - Go to Google and look up dating sites. Choose a first site to explore. Ask yourself questions: What sort of people post on this site? How old are they? Are they under thirty? Over fifty? Are they professionals? Athletes? The earthy-crunchy sort? Do you like what you see? Look at some individual profiles. Think about how you might write your profile. Spend two hours.

Day 2 - Check out two more dating sites. Follow Day One's steps. Spend two hours.

Day 3 - Choose two dating sites. Then, start writing your profile. Be honest and present yourself in a good light. Make your language come alive. Spend two hours.

Day 4 - Complete your profile. Ask someone you respect to read it. Hear her suggestions. Spend two hours.

Day 5 - Have someone take pictures of you. Make sure the pictures show you smiling. If this is done on a digital camera, review the pictures and decide which ones you like. Spend an hour.

Day 6 -Take your camera to a processing center. Have a CD made with the pictures. If possible, wait for your pictures and review them. Spend two hours.

Day 7- Upload your pictures onto the two dating sites you have chosen. Read over your profile, then publish it on both sites. Spend two hours.

End of Week 1 - Reward yourself for work well-done. Go to the movies or out for pizza.

Day 8 - Check out dating site number one to see if you've gotten any hits. If you have, think about responding. Look at other people's profiles. If you find someone of interest, wink or send an email. Spend two hours.

Day 9 - Check out dating site number two to see if anyone has winked at you. If they have, think about emailing the person. Look at other people's profiles. If you find someone appealing, wink. Look in your local newspaper for singles' activities. Choose an activity and plan on going. Spend two hours.

Day 10 - Check out your dating sites again for hits. Respond to those who have looked at you. Look at other people's profiles. Think about winking. Take your dog for a walk. If you see someone of interest walking a dog, let your dog's leash get tangled up with hers. If something comes of it, great. If not, apologize and walk away. Say "bad dog" to your pup then sneak him a treat. Spend two hours.

You get the idea.

The form I work with for "Realizing My Goals" is basic and divided into sections. I suggest you make copies of this form.

REALIZING MY GOAL FORM

WHAT IS MY GOAL?

_____
_____
_____
_____
_____
_____
_____
_____

HOW AM I GOING TO ACHIEVE MY GOAL?

_____
_____
_____
_____
_____
_____
_____
_____

WHAT OBSTACLES ARE IN THE WAY OF REACHING MY GOAL?

DO I PLAN TO ADDRESS MY OBSTACLES OR CHANGE THE SPECIFICS OF MY GOAL?

IF I AM GOING TO CHANGE MY SPECIFICS, WHAT WILL I CHANGE?

IF I WANT TO OVERCOME MY OBSTACLES, HOW AM I GOING TO DO SO?

_____
_____
_____
_____
_____
_____
_____

REALIZING MY GOAL - WEEKLY PLAN

WEEK _____ DAY ONE   HOW LONG WILL I SPEND ON IT? _____

WHAT WILL I DO TODAY IN AN EFFORT TO REACH MY GOAL?

_____
_____
_____
_____
_____
_____
_____

WEEK _____ DAY TWO   HOW LONG WILL I SPEND ON IT? _____

WHAT WILL I DO TODAY IN AN EFFORT TO REACH MY GOAL?

_____
_____
_____

_____
_____
_____
_____
_____
_____

WEEK _____ DAY THREE   HOW LONG WILL I SPEND ON IT? _____

WHAT WILL I DO TODAY IN AN EFFORT TO REACH MY GOAL?

_____
_____
_____
_____
_____
_____
_____

WEEK _____ DAY FOUR   HOW LONG WILL I SPEND ON IT? _____

WHAT WILL I DO TODAY IN AN EFFORT TO REACH MY GOAL?

_____
_____
_____
_____
_____
_____
_____

IF I COULD SNAP OUT OF IT, DON'T YOU THINK I WOULD?

WEEK _____ DAY FIVE   HOW LONG WILL I SPEND ON IT? _____

WHAT WILL I DO TODAY IN AN EFFORT TO REACH MY GOAL?

_____
_____
_____
_____
_____
_____
_____
_____

WEEK _____ DAY SIX   HOW LONG WILL I SPEND ON IT? _____

WHAT WILL I DO TODAY IN AN EFFORT TO REACH MY GOAL?

_____
_____
_____
_____
_____
_____
_____
_____

WEEK _____ DAY SEVEN   HOW LONG WILL I SPEND ON IT? _____

WHAT WILL I DO TODAY IN AN EFFORT TO REACH MY GOAL?

_____
_____
_____
_____

DON'T SET YOUR SIGHTS SHORT—GO AFTER EVERYTHING YOU WANT

You've set a goal and you are going after it. You're going to quit smoking or meet someone or lose weight or...This is great. Really great. But don't forget the even bigger stuff.

So many people I meet say they wish they had done things differently. They wish they had gone to college or graduate school or had children or traveled. When I ask them why they don't do now whatever it is they want to do, they usually say things like, "Oh, it's not possible. I'm too old," or, "I've got a family now, responsibilities, you know..."

You've only got one life. Go after what you want. Don't give in to your obstacles too quickly. Think outside the box. Perhaps you want to go back to college, but you have kids and a full-time job. Consider going to school at night or on weekends. Lots of colleges accommodate working people. Or consider an online degree. Suppose you've always wanted children, but you are forty-five and have never been married. That doesn't mean that you can't adopt a child. Maybe you won't be able to work with a traditional adoption agency, but you may be able to adopt through social services. There are children out there waiting to be adopted, children who might love being yours.

Don't give up because things are hard. If you can't accomplish your goal one way, try another way.

Think creatively. Don't be afraid to ask for help.

Here are three stories of people who went after the big stuff. While details have been changed to assure confidentiality, the stories are true.

Jackson was very smart, but didn't believe in himself. He had quit high school when he was sixteen. Jackson loved animals. At one time he had wanted to be a veterinarian, but he had never pursued it. At the age of twenty-four, Jackson was supporting himself by house-sitting and walking dogs. He had friends, but most of them drank and did drugs. He had few good supports. He hardly ever talked to his parents; long ago they had grown tired of his behavior. Every so often, when things got bad, he cut his arms.

After one of his girlfriends left him, Jackson became severely depressed. He spent two days in bed and contemplated suicide. But he knew he didn't want to die. What Jackson realized, however, was that he wasn't living the way he wanted to be living. He decided it was time to make changes. Jackson always had wanted to be a veterinarian. He knew that if he was going to pursue this goal, he needed to do so now. Without a wife or kids, he could afford to be poor for a while.

Although he was scared, Jackson enrolled in a GED course. Two months later, he breezed through his high school equivalency test. It was a good ego boost. From there, Jackson went over to the local community college and met with an advisor. He explained to her that he wanted to be a veterinarian, but that he had no money and didn't think his parents would help. She directed him to the appropriate people and he received financial aid. He attended this community college for two years, supporting himself by walking dogs and house-sitting. He kept a 3.92 average. In his second year of community college, he applied to a university. He was accepted and received a scholarship. While at the university, he kept a straight A average. In his senior year, he applied to a well-respected veterinary school and was accepted, all tuition paid.

The last time I spoke to Jackson, he had finished his last year of veterinary school. He had just adopted a parrot who had been left at the school's veterinary clinic. He loved his work.

If I were a betting person, I would guess that Jackson is in veterinary practice today. I would also guess that his office is full of some very happy animals.

Here's another true story, with only the details changed.

Paul grew up poor, with a young, single mother who had tuberculosis and was in and out of hospitals. She never told him anything about his father. When Paul would ask about his dad, his mother would say, "There's nothing to tell you." Unfortunately, Paul's mother died when he was thirteen.

After his mother's death, Paul went to live with some distant relatives. They were elderly and never got too involved with the boy. Paul was lost. He had no sense of his roots.

At eighteen, Paul tried to enlist in the army. He was told he needed his birth certificate.

Paul didn't know where he had been born. He sent a letter to the county office for the town where he and his mother had lived. He gave them his name, his mother's name, and his date of birth.

Weeks later, he received a notice that no match was found. He expanded his search to numerous surrounding counties. A month and a half later, his birth certificate arrived. With it, was the name of his father.

Now Paul was intrigued. He wanted to go into the service, but that could wait. He had a quest: he wanted to find his father.

Paul remembered the names of some towns his mother had mentioned—places where she had lived as a child and a teenager. He went to a couple of these towns and looked around. He searched the phone books. There were no listings of anyone with his father's last name.

He continued searching. In the third town, there was a hardware store bearing his father's last name. He tried his hand here. He hit gold dust, sort of. He learned that this hardware store had been owned previously by a man who bore his father's first and last name. The new owner had bought the store from him. Months after the papers were signed, the man had died. The new owner didn't know if the man had any family in the area.

Paul's surname was not common. And his father's first name was particularly unusual. The store's previous owner had to be his father. And sadly, Paul would never have the chance to know him.

The sadness didn't last too long. Maybe there were family members.

Paul continued his search and extended it into surrounding towns. Then counties. Months later, he found a man who shared his father's surname. It turned out to be his father's brother.

The brother confirmed that Paul's father was dead. But his father had never been married, the uncle said. He didn't have any children.

The uncle was wary. Who was this boy? What did he want?

At first, the uncle denied knowing Paul's mother. However, after a while, the uncle came clean. He said he did know Paul's mother. She had gone to high school with his brother and him. Paul's father had gone out with her once or twice. Paul's uncle had thought she had moved out of town. He knew nothing about his brother having a son. He was sure his brother had known nothing about it either.

At first, the relationship between Paul and the uncle was strained. Why had Paul come to find him, the uncle wondered. Was Paul after something beside his roots? Was it all legitimate?

Paul persisted. The uncle came to believe him. And in him. A relationship formed. Then a bond.

At age twenty-five, Paul married. His uncle was the best man at his wedding.

Paul had found his roots.

And yet another story.

Years ago, I was a teacher. In one of my classes there was a very quiet Cambodian boy named Sovann. I didn't know much about him.

One day, in response to an assignment I had given, I learned Sovann's story. I can tell it almost verbatim today, twenty-five years later.

Sovann had grown up in Cambodia. His father was a very smart man and a general in the army. His uncle was a doctor. As a boy, Sovann had enjoyed sitting with his uncle, looking through his medical books. His uncle explained many medical procedures to Sovann.

Then the Khmer Rouge seized power in Cambodia. Their plan was to wipe out the country's intelligentsia.

At age nine, Sovann was forced to watch as his father and uncle were lined up and executed by the Khmer Rouge. Then he, his mother, and siblings were taken to various collective farms. Sovann and two of his brothers were taken to a farm and forced to work very long hours: plowing, hoeing, building irrigation works. For a long period, each boy on the farm was fed one banana or a bit of rice gruel a day. Many died of starvation.

One day, Sovann was working in the fields. He heard screaming. Seeing that the guard was asleep, he chanced it, followed the sound, and found a young woman giving birth. He remembered enough from his uncle's textbooks that he was able to cut the baby's umbilical cord using the sharp edge of a rock.

Sovann knew that the rocks around camp contained iron. He also knew that iron strengthened the immune system.

Knowing that he and the others were very weak, Sovann took every opportunity to scrape iron from the rocks. He hid the pieces of iron in his clothing and snuck them into camp. He gave the pieces to the boys and instructed them to grind them as much as possible, mix with water, and drink. He told them it would help build their strength.

Eventually, Sovann and his two brothers were able to escape. They had to walk across Cambodia, avoiding land mines and the carcasses of the dead. They made it to the border. Months later, an aid worker reunited them with an uncle. They learned their mother had died.

Over the next two years, Sovann's brothers died, likely from diseases they had picked up in the camp. Three years after their escape, Sovann and his uncle made the voyage to America. They settled in Washington, D.C., where Sovann's uncle became a cab driver. Sovann, age twelve, procured a job landscaping for a professor of history at a local university. On a rainy night, Sovann's uncle was killed, his cab hit by another vehicle. The professor and his wife took Sovann in. They moved to Massachusetts where I met him.

The last time I saw Sovann was at his high school graduation. He explained to me that although his high school grades were good, he was to going to attend a post-high school program to improve his English. He wanted his English to be fluent for college. After college, he was going to attend medical school. "I will do my residency in internal medicine," he said. "Then I will return to Cambodia and help my people."

Go after what you want, no matter how hard it is. Live your life.

CHAPTER SEVEN

WEAR YOUR COGNITIVE HAT

I KNEW SOMETHING WAS MISSING IN the treatment of depression. After all, as a therapist, I saw my clients come in weekly, bruised and beaten by their depression, only to leave fifty minutes later, with restored hope and a willingness to continue fighting.

But the gains made in weekly sessions seldom lasted.

Week after week clients arrived, as battered as they had been the week before. When I asked if they had worked on the exercises or approaches we had discussed in therapy, the responses were usually, "No, I meant to…but" or, "I forgot" or, "It was a hard week."

I had to ask: Why didn't the momentum begun in therapy carry through?

The answer was simple.

Fighting depression is extremely hard work. To beat depression, people have to do so much. They have to stay busy, go out, and try to connect with other people. They have to give of themselves to people and to goals bigger than they. They have to start liking and believing in themselves. They have to confront what they don't like about themselves, decide what they want to change, create a game plan to make this change happen, and work on the plan daily. And they have to do all this with the burden of depression upon them, having little energy, less motivation, and the belief that things will never get better.

Even the idea of the work is overwhelming.

I wondered if there was something out there that would make the process easier.

I thought of Jake, a client with whom I once worked.

Jake, a young man of twenty-four, had lived a very hard life. He had grown up poor, with an aunt and uncle who were disabled. He had graduated from high school, but had not been a great student. He never went to college. "All I ever wanted to do was fly," he said. At eighteen, he had thought of joining the Air Force, but felt he couldn't leave his aunt and uncle to fend for themselves.

When I met Jake, he had a girlfriend of two years and a baby who was almost a year old. He had a decent job working for an import-export company. He liked it O.K., but he didn't make much money. His job was close to the airport and often, while driving to work, he would see the planes flying in. That was his favorite part of his job.

Jake was proud of the fact that he worked hard and was able to support his girlfriend and baby and help his aunt and uncle who lived nearby. Recently, his uncle had suffered a stroke.

Shortly after Jake and I began working together, I learned that a local community college had begun a two-year aviation program. Students could learn to fly in this program. The program wasn't very expensive, financial aid was available, and one did not have to be a great student to get in. I encouraged Jake to look into it.

At first, Jake was thrilled. "Oh God," he said. "I could really do this." He made an appointment with an admissions counselor at the school.

Jake learned that the school offered a very flexible schedule. There were daytime, evening, and weekend hours. He could go part-time, take longer than two years to finish, and get financial aid. He probably would have to add on a second job to afford the tuition, but he could make it happen. Jake decided to go. He was ecstatic.

The next time I saw Jake, his mood had deflated. The plan wasn't realistic, he said. If he worked two jobs, he wouldn't have enough time for his girlfriend or his baby. How would he get his schoolwork done while working two jobs? School was always hard for him. "Money will be really tight," he said. He and his girlfriend would have to give up things. He said he still had to give money to his aunt and uncle.

We spent the session considering the obstacles. While not easy, each could be overcome. He could work extra time at his job and still go to school. He might not have as much time with his girlfriend or baby as he had now, but he would see them. He believed their relationship was strong enough to withstand the reduction in time. He could get his work done. The community college offered lots of tutoring. He could get help in the subjects that were difficult. In two years' time, with a career in aviation, he would be able to offer his girlfriend and baby a better life. And what a great thing it would be for his self-esteem if he actually became what he always wanted to become.

He was flying on his own steam when he left the session.

The third time I saw Jake he had started taking classes. "It's hard," he said. The writing course was tough. He was tired. His girlfriend was annoyed at him. He would have to cut therapy to twice a month, he said. The co-pays were too much. He wasn't in the best of moods.

By the time he left the session, however, he was able to say that he could and would continue on with school. He was going to be a pilot.

I never saw Jake again. Although I called him several times, he never returned my calls.

I could be wrong, but I assume that he did not continue on with school. It probably got to be too much.

But the questions lingered. Why was it that when we talked, he felt he could muster the strength to tackle the aviation program, but when he was out in the world, it became too much? Was it that we hadn't been realistic enough when considering the obstacles? Was the program too expensive? Were there not enough hours in the day? Did Jake lack the ability to do the work? I don't believe it was any of these. Juggling work, school, and family would certainly have been difficult. But he could have done it.

I think what was missing was having an impartial someone who believed in him when he wasn't in therapy. Someone who wanted Jake to succeed, even if it meant that life, temporarily, would be more difficult. Someone who could say "yes" when Jake said "no." Someone who would say, "You can do this" when he thought he couldn't. Someone who would challenge his automatic thoughts when his thoughts were negative. Someone who would prod him on when he felt like giving up. What he needed was a "therapist sort-of" on his shoulder.

GET A MOOD COACH

A "mood coach" is how I refer to an acquaintance/friend/relative who wants for you what you want for you and cares about you enough to work with you for one half to one hour weekly. A mood coach is someone who will sit down with you and listen as you read your daily, chronicled, automatic thoughts aloud. He/she will call you on it when you sabotage yourself, hold you accountable when you give up, and prod you onward and give you kudos when you are doing well.

It is not necessary for a mood coach to be a trained therapist or even to be schooled in psychology. What is necessary is that the mood coach be committed to you and have your best interest, as defined by you, in mind.

Let's consider how a mood coach might have worked with Jake, the client described above.

If Jake had committed himself to the mood-changing plan described in this book, he would have already been recording his daily, automatic thoughts and his talk-back to these thoughts. It is these automatic thoughts and rebuttals that Jake would be sharing with his mood coach.

The first automatic thought Jake might have shared with his mood coach would likely have been written soon after he started aviation school.

"I can't do this."

Jake then would have shared his talk-back to this thought.

"I can do this; I'm just not sure I want to."

After hearing Jake's automatic thought and his talk-back to his thought, the mood coach might have commented, "Is that true, Jake? You really don't want to be a pilot?"

Jake then would have answered.

"Well no, it's not true. I do want to be a pilot."

Wanting more information, the mood coach would have encouraged Jake to go on.

"Why don't you read your next thought and talk-back," the mood coach would have said.

"I don't have the money to go to school and keep everybody going," Jake would have read.

Then Jake would have shared his talk-back to this thought.

"Well, I can make the money and make it work, but it's just so hard."

At this point, the mood coach would have challenged Jake.

"Jake, I guess you have to decide if it's worth it to you to work your butt off for two years to get what you want. What you've always wanted."

And so on…

See how the mood coach would have called Jake on his self-sabotaging thoughts? See how he would have kept him on target?

A mood coach is your 'therapist-sort of' when you are not with your therapist. And keep this in mind. A mood coach does not have his/her own agenda. A mood coach wants for you what you want for you. Always.

So where do you find a mood coach?

A spouse, girlfriend, or boyfriend is out; their lives are too intertwined with yours and objectivity is too difficult. Can parents be mood coaches? In my opinion, some can, but most can't.

For some people, finding a mood coach is no harder than looking to the homes where they grew up or the hometowns where they went to school. It might be the brothers or sisters who always believed in them or the best friends they've had since third grade.

If you don't have a sibling with whom you are close or a friend of twenty years, don't despair. A new friend with whom you've shared feelings also might be a good option. Choose someone who has allowed you to see that she also is struggling. Think of it this way. A mood coach is beneficial for both of you. She can help you and you can help her. When you approach a new friend to be a mood coach, start by saying that she may not be at all interested and that's totally O.K. Then explain that you are on a roll to accomplish what you want to in life, and you are done sabotaging yourself. Explain that you've been exploring a technique in which you chronicle your automatic thoughts and your talkback to these thoughts. Explain that a key part of the technique is to find an impartial party by whom you can run your thoughts. Give a few examples. Make clear that you'll be happy to be her mood coach as well. Specify that you are talking about no more than an hour a week and that if it doesn't work for her, she can pull out. Again, reiterate, that if she is uninterested, it's totally O.K.

A mood coach doesn't have to be a friend, even a new one. You also can look for a mood coach in the acquaintances you encounter in day-to-day activities. Have you talked to someone at the gym, in class, or at a play group who seems to be struggling? If so, go out on a limb. You might find a coach and a friend as well.

For those who do not have close family, good friends, many acquaintances, or daily activities, finding a mood coach takes more work. But don't give up. You can find one.

In fact, there are lots of possibilities.

Priests, ministers, and rabbis are good options. These people enjoy helping their members succeed and are trained to help. However, if you approach your clergyman, he may or may not have the weekly time to help. If he does not, don't take it personally. Depression groups also are good places to find mood coaches. NAMI, the National Alliance on Mental Illness, your local hospital, or your local newspaper will likely have a listing of depression groups. The advantage in looking for a mood coach in an already existing depression group is that once you explain the process, the other person quickly will see the sense of a mood coach. If you don't find any groups in your area, consider starting your own mood group. You could do so by creating a flyer about the group and giving it to your therapist, doctor, or local mental health clinic. Once you gather people who are struggling with depression, you can explain the theory behind having a mood coach. Then, within the group, you can partner up.

REALITY-TEST YOUR NEGATIVE THOUGHTS

Cognitive techniques help you question and change your thinking. Recording your automatic thoughts and talking back to them may be the most important and effective cognitive technique. But there are others.

Sometimes it's hard to know if your negative thoughts are realistic. This is particularly true if your thoughts involve others. To check things out, you need to reality-test your thoughts. Maybe you think you're a burden to others. Are you? Or is this just you, doing what you do best, sucker-punching yourself?

Maybe you think your husband would be happier if you left him. Would he? Maybe you think your grown children don't want you around. Is this true?

To know the truth, you have to ask for it. Look it squarely in the big blues. No averting your face. No hiding your head under your coat.

If you are going to ask people to tell you the truth, you have to tell them that you want the truth. And that you are ready and willing to deal with it. Before you do so, however, you have to know that this is a fact. Can you deal with the truth? Have you grown enough to know that whatever the truth is, you will be better off knowing it?

Does your husband want you to leave? Ask him. If he says yes, it will hurt. But at some point, you will be proud of yourself for caring enough about you to get out of a loveless relationship. If he says no, you will feel loved. You will realize that you have been punishing yourself without cause and you will work at stopping this behavior.

Do the same for your other thoughts that involve people. Facing the answers will allow you to grow. Ask your grown kids if they want you around. Maybe they'll tell you that they hate it when you nag them so much and hate it when you are critical, but yeah, it wouldn't be the same if you weren't around. Maybe their saying this will allow you to see your kids for the adults they are, adults who are entitled to make their own choices and their own mistakes. And maybe, by seeing this, what was once a frayed relationship will become a beautifully repaired one. Suppose your kids say, "No, we don't want you around." This will be painful, but you will know that space between you and your kids is necessary, at least for the time being. If you ask them why it is that they don't want you around and really listen to their answers, you may be able to do the work necessary to repair the relationship.

Maybe your thoughts don't involve others, but, rather, a perception of yourself.

Perhaps you think you are too flabby or too soft. A guy without muscle. Are you? Is there someone you can ask and get an honest answer? If so, ask her. Again, preface this by saying you want the truth. And mean it. If there are no friends or family to ask, ask your doctor or trainer at the gym. Then ask for suggestions as to what to do to gain muscle and definition. Maybe that six-pack is attainable.

Suppose you think you are ugly. This is a difficult one. There is no such thing as absolute beauty. Beauty is a perception, perceived by the one who is looking. However, even the loveliest can enhance her looks. So try asking your question a different way. Approach a friend or family member and say that you want to enhance your looks and are looking for suggestions. Again, the trick is to ask honestly. Otherwise, it is a setup for the person you ask.

SAYING POSITIVE THINGS TO YOURSELF

You are a master at beating yourself up. But you are lousy at telling yourself anything positive. No one is all good or all bad. You are not the definition of "rotten" because you cheated on your boyfriend. You are the same person who is nice to the little kids at the walk-in clinic.

It doesn't matter if you think your bad qualities outnumber your good. Start acknowledging your good qualities. Tell yourself what you do well. Then write them down.

Here are some examples of positive statements. Review them for ideas, and then write your own.

I am funny.
I succeed when I try.
I think for myself.
I am kind to animals.
I am a good person.
I have a good heart.
I have a good voice.
I am smart.
I am a good woodworker.
I am good with little kids.
I am a good mechanic.

Write each of your positive statements on index cards. Make two cards for each positive statement. When new positive statements come to mind, write them down. Keep one copy of the index cards somewhere private. Post the other cards where you are sure to see them. Read the cards aloud to yourself at least three times a day. After some practice, start reading these statements to yourself while looking in the mirror.

Remember, we believe the things we do about ourselves because that's what we've been told. It doesn't matter who does the telling. So start telling yourself all that is good about you.

IT'S EITHER A ZEBRA OR A POSTER

In the classic cognitive behavioral work *Feeling Good*, author David Burns provides his readers with ten common cognitive distortions. A cognitive distortion is an error in thinking, a twisting of what should be very plain. Think of a balloon master, who takes an ordinary pink balloon from the hands of a five-year-old and, before her eyes, turns it into a miniature French poodle.

While I don't think it necessary to address all the cognitive distortions, in my opinion, there are a few that do particular damage. It is these I will address.

I refer to the first cognitive distortion as A Zebra or A Poster thinking-or what is known in cognitive literature as All or Nothing thinking. I call it this because a zebra and a poster have nothing in common with each other, in fact, they are entirely different entities, which is pretty much how people with this thinking see things. To these folks, things are defined in absolutes, one thing is the polar opposite of another. The muted gray that almost always exists between black and white cannot be seen. A current friend "is awesome, completely awesome," a once-friend is a "shit, always was, always will be," and a Mustang is "the best car ever made, hands down."

People with A Zebra or A Poster thinking also categorize the responses to their behaviors or actions in extremes: either everyone they meet likes them or they have no friends; either they get callbacks from every acting audition for which they have tried out or they are forever relegated to the lighting crews; either they are catapulted to the top of every position they hold or they are complete failures.

People with this thinking act as if their good and bad qualities, their successes and failures, have nothing to do with each other. In fact, we can only succeed if we know failure. Failure is a teaching tool. It shows us how to do things better, how to grow.

Learn to tackle this problematic thinking. Suppose you go for a job interview and are not offered the position. Jumping to, "I fail at everything," is inaccurate. No one fails at everything. Did you fail at eating breakfast this morning? Did you fail fourth grade? Did you fail at falling in love for the first time? Resorting to A Zebra or A Poster thinking is self-sabotaging and does little to help you grow. Rather, ask yourself what might have prevented you from being offered the job. Did you present yourself positively? Were you confident enough? Were your references the best they could be? Was the job a good fit for you? If the answer to each of these questions is yes, consider calling your interviewer for feedback. Explain that you want to know why you weren't considered for the position. Do so politely and honestly, then thank her for her response.

Taking this step requires courage, but the learning opportunities are huge.

Then, take what you learn and do something about it. Improve what you need to improve.

Here is a true story—one close to my heart and straight from my child. I had nothing to do with it.

When my oldest daughter, Alexa, was in sixth grade, she wanted to be a cheerleader. Truly wanted to be a cheerleader. So she did what kids do when they have this desire. She tried out for the team.

Now, in sixth grade, the word "tryout" is a misnomer. Kids tryout and if they show up, they make the team. Alexa showed up. She was on the team.

Most of the kids on the team, Alexa included, did not know much about cheerleading. The girls went to the games and entertained the crowd. They had spirit. That was it.

The season was going nicely.

Then talk of an exhibition team came up. It was a new concept to the kids. If they formed an exhibition team, they could compete against other teams in big gymnasiums to the roar of huge audiences. The kids loved the idea.

The coach held tryouts for this team. But unbeknownst to the kids, the rules of "tryouts" were different this time. While there were twenty-four kids on the cheerleading team, only twenty could be on the exhibition team. Four eleven-year-old girls would have to be cut.

The tryouts were held on a Thursday night. I was not around. I worked at the hospital on Thursday nights. Worse, I didn't know the tryouts were taking place.

Arriving home from work that night, I found my daughter hysterical. She hadn't made the exhibition team. She explained that the tryouts had been held in the gymnasium, in front of a crowd of parents and kids. The names of the kids who had made the team had been read aloud, leaving the four who didn't make the team to cringe in front of everyone.

My mama bear came out. I berated the cheerleading organization with every four letter word I knew. In true stick-it-out fashion, I told Alexa to quit the team.

"No," she said.

I wasn't going to allow my child to be embarrassed, I said. I stood on my ever-handy soapbox and spewed about how sports are meant to build children's self-esteem. I commiserated on what an awful experience this must have been for an eleven-year-old child. I decided that my daughter's self-esteem had been destroyed.

The next day I cried to my boss, who just happened to be a football coach and a very sweet man.

"They've destroyed her," I said.

"I don't think so," he said. "Kids are resilient. You'll be surprised."

I didn't listen. I told Alexa to quit the team. Again.

"No," she said. "Just because I didn't make the team doesn't mean I can't be a good cheerleader."

Alexa continued with the cheerleading team. She went to all the exhibition meets. Instead of performing on the mat, she waved hand-held signs that read, "Go girls. You're awesome." She didn't say a word about being sidelined.

For the next two years, Alexa sat in on the practices of a well-known, competitive cheerleading team. She was not a member of that team, but she was allowed to learn and practice along with these girls.

By the time Alexa was thirteen, she had become a competent enough cheerleader to join a competitive team. Twice a week, she traveled one and a half hours to do three hours of push-ups, jumping jacks, and cheerleading stunts.

As a freshman in high school, Alexa tried out for the school's cheerleading team. In high school, tryouts mean something. She was one of three freshman girls to make the team. By her junior year, Alexa was elected cheerleading captain.

In her senior year, Alexa and her teammates were the first cheerleading team ever from their school to make it to the national cheerleading competitions held at Universal Studios in Orlando, Florida.

The moral of the story: If you want something badly enough, don't give up. Do what it takes. Persevere. And don't listen to your mother.

You're setting yourself up for failure if A Zebra or A Poster is your way of seeing the world. Things are not all one way or another. Ask parents how many times a week they fail at parenting. Ask any couple how many times a week they fail at their relationship.

A Zebra or A Poster thinking is a trap. It lets you off the hook. It prevents you from growing.

HALF-EMPTY PHENOMENON

Is the glass half-full or half-empty? Of course, a glass that is filled half-way is both. However, people who struggle with the Half-Empty Phenomenon cannot see the glass as half-full.

For example, suppose you live in a coastal town that was just hit by a hurricane. Your yard was flooded and your flower beds and vegetable garden ruined. But your house was spared. As a person who sees the world as half-empty, all you can think of are the problems in your yard. When a neighbor stops by and comments on how lucky you are that your house was spared, you want to smack her. "What is she? An idiot?" you think. "Doesn't she see my yard?"

Why is it that you only can see the negative?

I believe those who struggle with this phenomenon are afraid of being disappointed. They believe that if they don't expect much, they can't lose much. One of my clients calls this "pre-disastering." He says that if he thinks about all that can go wrong in any given situation, he'll be ready. If something good happens, it will be like he's won his own personal lottery.

People with the Half-Empty Phenomenon feel they are being proactive, preparing themselves for the worst, in much the same way as the people who built underground cellars in case of nuclear war believed they were preparing for disaster. I think those with this phenomenon deprive themselves of everyday joy.

Let's go back to our earlier example. The hurricane has destroyed your flower beds and vegetable garden, but left your home intact.

Suppose you concentrated on the positive. Suppose you said to yourself, "I'm so lucky that no water came into my house. Water would have destroyed my furniture, turned things moldy. Who knows what insurance would have covered? I don't like that my gardens were destroyed, but I can redo them. Maybe next year I'll plant an even bigger vegetable garden."

Thinking like this would do much to boost your spirits and it would not make the replanting of your garden any more difficult. In fact, it would give you more energy to plan for a bigger and better garden.

REFRAMING

Sometimes, good things come out of lousy situations. Recently, I pulled out my back. I believe it was because I carried three full gallons of paint at one time. Rather than carrying one in each hand and coming back for the third, I stubbornly insisted on carrying them all at once, ambling out of the store, lopsided. For several days after, I barely could move. All this forced me to go to the doctor, which led to an x-ray, which, in turn, caused me to discover that I have a problem with the density of the bones in my spine. Not a life-threatening condition, but one with the potential to sideline me if I don't do something about it.

Even though I've always been relatively thin, I tend to carry all my weight in my stomach. Sometimes, after eating a meal, complete with bread and dessert, my stomach, with an intestinal mind of its own, juts out like a left-open bureau drawer. Of course, I don't like this. I also realized that my stomach was putting a strain on my back, but I figured it was one of those things I had to live with.

However, realizing I had to improve matters with my back (and my bones), I bought a book on bone health. I expected to read about the need to drink more milk and eat more cheese, but this wasn't the case. Rather, the authors made a surprising claim, supported with lots of research: a diet rich in fruits, vegetables, nuts, seeds, and very few processed foods, coupled with walking, could turn lousy bone health into pretty robust bone health. Anyway, the long and short of it is that I started eating a lot more vegetables and fruits and substituted unadulterated chocolate chips for my previously very processed cookies and brownies. It was a eureka experience. My former left-open-bureau-drawer-of-a-stomach began to stay closed. So a bad situation turned into a learning opportunity, which, in turn, caused me to change my behavior.

Reframing means putting a positive spin on things. The positive spin to pulling out my back is that it caused me to discover a life-altering way for me and my stomach to be friends. In fact, I'll go so far as to say that pulling out my back likely will add years to my life. How's that for a reframe?

"LIFE SUCKS" AND OTHER SUCH "IT'S NOT FAIR" THINKING

Some people carry around the attitude "Life Sucks" like a backpack. They wear it daily. They stuff it with their experiences, past and present. It's like they think life owes them more.

For most of us, life gives us plenty. The rest is up to us.

You say you want love, adventure, a good job, and money? Then go for it.

You don't have what you want? Then fix it, work on it, change it.

Take more time to appreciate the world. Stand in awe at the blue of the sky, at cherry trees that blossom in spring, at sunflowers that poke their heads skyward in summer, at human minds capable of conceptualizing the galaxies. Be thankful for your health, for shelter from the cold. Be thankful that you are able to witness the magic of existence.

Learn from those who suffer greatly—young girls sold into the sex trade, refugee families whose only windows are the open spaces between flimsy pieces of rusted barbed wire, victims of earthquakes and tsunamis whose homes and lives are reduced to rubble, parents forced to relive the horror of their children's abductions and murders. Learn from what some of these people have done with their pain—turning what could be endless self-pity into tireless work, so that one more person, one more family, may be spared what they have had to endure.

Forget "Life Sucks." Take up a new battle cry. How about: "Life—Always Worth the Fight."

SEARCH FOR MEANING

Happy people have meaning and purpose in their lives. But where do these come from? Are we born with the knowledge of what we are meant to do?

I believe the answer is no. Most of us discover what is meaningful to us by living our lives. Many who are drawn to the field of mental health have struggled with depression or anxiety. Many who are drawn to teaching have had their lives turned around by a wonderful teacher. Some very successful business people have struggled with poverty.

Some of us flounder in our search for meaning. We reach forty and fifty years old and haven't an inkling. We wait for a purpose to reveal itself. But what if it never does? Is it O.K. for us to reach out and find our own purpose?

I think it is more than O.K.

Perhaps it's our job in life to find a purpose.

But how do we know what purpose to choose if it doesn't choose us?

Start by thinking about those people who you most admire. What is it they do? Do they help rid war-torn countries of land mines? Do they raise money for orphanages? Do they work to save the great apes or the elephants? Do they run for office, play cello, or raise sweet children?

Think about the things that make life brilliant for you, the things for which you are willing to really fight. Consider the needs out there. Then, remember that a single person can make a difference in the world.

One of my clients was lost. She had been married, but that had ended. She had hoped to marry again, but hadn't met anyone. She had no children or siblings. She saw her parents occasionally. She had friends, but most were married with children. They were busy. Due to a disability, my client worked only part-time. She cried a lot and felt that her life lacked meaning. She loved animals.

One night, driving on a busy road in downtown Boston, she saw a dog about to cross the road. Cars were everywhere.

She immediately pulled her car to the curb and beckoned to the animal. The dog came right to her. The dog was thin, as if she hadn't eaten for some time and had no collar or identification. My client put the dog in her car and took her to an animal shelter. The dog was sick and needed care. My client paid for the care herself and advertised for anyone who might have lost a dog. She got no response. A month later she adopted the dog and named her Lucky.

My client began thinking about all the dogs and cats out there. Many were sick and starving. She began driving around, searching for stray animals. She found colonies of feral cats and began feeding them. The money for the cat food was money my client earned herself. She learned about no-kill shelters. Some months later, she captured her first feral cats, brought them to shelters, had them neutered and given shots, and returned them to the wild. She sought out stray dogs. She took them to the shelters as well, where they were neutered, given medical treatment, and put up for adoption.

To date, my client has saved many dogs and hundreds of cats.

Her life took on meaning.

Another of my clients was well-to-do. He was a CEO for a flourishing company. He had a wife he loved, great kids, a beautiful house, cars, and the ability to travel all over the world, but he struggled with depression. His life seemed empty. One day he was talking to a coworker who had adopted three siblings from abroad. One of the siblings had a cleft palate. The coworker and his wife were pursuing the surgery that would correct the defect and allow the child's beautiful face to be seen. As my client got to know this man, he learned about the hardships these children had endured when they were young and about the poverty in their country, the lack of medical care, and the prejudice against anyone with a facial disfiguration.

My client donated money to an organization fighting poverty in that country. He also donated to another group that helped children with cleft palates obtain the surgery they so needed. He spread the word to others he knew and they also donated. Now, every year, instead of giving Christmas presents, he and his family donate the money they would spend to these two organizations. He also has taken on several other causes. He is a much happier man.

How do you start fighting depression? Do something for someone else. Help someone who is in need.

You will see that a key activity in the mood-changing plan is to volunteer your services. In Chapter Eight, I discuss the specifics on volunteering. For now, spend your time honing in on the causes that matter to you. When you are ready to volunteer, you will know where to offer your services.

The satisfaction that comes from making a difference in another's life is powerful.

DREAM UP THE GUSTO

It's your life. Grab it. Shake it. Do what you want to do.

Think about it. What will make your life a life worth living? What have you always wanted to do? What would you have done if you weren't too scared, too busy, too practical or…?

"But I'm already forty," you say. "I'm already sixty."

Who cares? What will make you say, "I gave this life all I got, then I gave it more."

Do you want to sky dive? Ride a mule down the Grand Canyon? Help finance an orphanage? Backpack through Tibet? Live a year in Mexico? Save horses who are about to be slaughtered? Study painting in Paris? Fight poverty? Find a partner? Write a book?

I heard a story on the radio about a woman who went sky-diving for her birthday. It wouldn't have been much of a story had she not been in her eighties. I know of a man in my town who climbed the second tallest mountain in Alaska. He was eighty-one.

Don't say you can't do what you want because of money. There are ways around a lack of money. But you can't have it all. You may need to give up something to get another. If you want to travel, you may need to get a second job. Maybe you need to give up the idea of staying in hotels and opt for staying in campgrounds or hostels instead. Maybe you can volunteer somewhere abroad, then stay a little longer to see the area.

Think about whatever it is you want to do. Research it. See yourself doing it. Think about the pros, the cons. Think about what you will gain. Think about what you will have to give up. Then, remember, life is short, like the season of the apple. Take a bite. Live fully.

JOURNALING

It takes soul-searching to discover what matters to you, to find the qualities you like and don't like about yourself. It takes more soul searching to understand why you believe what you do about yourself.

Journaling is a great soul-searching technique.

You don't need to be a good writer to journal. You don't have to like writing. You do need to make a commitment to the process. It's a commitment to learning about you.

Start by deciding that the process is worthwhile. Understand that you will be learning about you, about the big and little things, the things that make you unique, the things that stand in your way.

Begin by buying yourself a journal. It doesn't have to be fancy. A notebook is fine. Label it "Journal." Keep it specifically for this task. If it is important for you to have your journal be private, label it "Private." If you don't think the people around you will respect your request for privacy, consider buying a journal with a lock.

Then, choose a certain time of day, the number of days per week that you will write, and the amount of time per day that you will commit to this process.

Don't worry if you don't have a topic. Write about anything.

Start with what happened that day. Or pose a daily question.

Use your five senses: sight, sound, taste, touch, and smell as starting points. Close your eyes and remember a smell—any smell: cookies just out of the oven, hamburgers on a grill, a newly cut Christmas tree, a puppy's breath. What memories do these smells conjure? Write about them.

Think about familiar sounds: rain hitting the roof, the burst of firecrackers, a thunderstorm, the church choir, a dog's bark. Let these memories take you where they will.

Think about things you have touched: beach sand, a soft comforter, a pine needle, the wood of a church pew, a cat's fur, your mother's hair. Go with it.

Think about sights you have experienced: a brightly lit city skyline, a policeman's uniform, a movie theatre marquee, a lifeguard stand, a deer. Where do these things take you?

Think about tastes: buttered popcorn, pizza bought from a vendor on the boardwalk, your grandmother's spaghetti, cotton candy, Rocky Road ice cream. Let the triggers take you for a ride.

Holidays are another good starting point. Think about Christmas, the Fourth of July, Thanksgiving, your birthday. You can jumpstart your memories by remembering where you were on these days. What did you eat? Who was there?

Think about the people who were important in your life: your grandparents, your uncles, your best friend, the first girl you kissed.

Think about your animals: the dog that slept in your bed, the cat who sat in your lap, the parrot who said, "Night-Night." How did you feel when you were with them?

Some people say their minds go blank when they try to write. If this is true for you, start by making scribbles on the paper. The point is to get the momentum going.

Some of your triggered memories may be painful. You need to decide if you can handle these memories by yourself. Being flooded by long-repressed memories can be overwhelming and dangerous.

Explore, but know when to ask for help.

VISUALIZATION

When you imagine a scene in your head, it comes alive. Suppose you imagine yourself on a beach. In your mind's eye, you see yourself in a bikini, lying on a towel. Perhaps your book is nearby, whatever current novel you are reading. The sun is shining, the day blue, and the water calm. As you look around, you see other people on the beach. Maybe there is a group of guys nearby. Maybe three of the guys are playing Frisbee. Maybe one of these guys is checking you out.

When you visualize something, it feels real. So it makes sense to use visualization as practice for the real thing.

Think about the things you have wanted for so long. Then, put your visualization strategies to work to help you achieve these goals.

Suppose you are shy. Suppose you'd love to walk into a party and talk to someone you don't know, but the very thought of this terrifies you. Try visualizing it. Imagine the party. What does the room look like? What is the lighting like? What music is playing? Look around and see the people. How are they dressed? How old are they? Listen in on their conversations. What are they talking about? Then visualize yourself walking up to a group and saying, "Hi." Imagine the woman on the end looking at you and saying, "Hello." Go further. Imagine introducing yourself. "I'm Cathy Mullin. I only know one person here." Imagine a few of the people laughing, not at you, but with you. Imagine one of the guys saying, "I don't know anybody." Hear everybody laugh. Then imagine one of the women saying, "I work with a man who is friends with the guy giving this party." Then listen as you yourself say, "That's how I got here too. One of my friends from work was invited. And she invited me."

Take a minute to pay attention to how you feel. Notice that as the visualization progressed, you began to feel accepted by the group and thus more relaxed.

Try another visualization. Visualize the same party, but give it a different twist. Imagine you walk into the party and see a crowd of smiling, talking people. You don't recognize anyone. Close to you is a woman standing by herself. You walk over and stand next to her.

"Hi," you say.
"Hi," she says.
"Looks like a nice party," you say.
"Yea," she says.
"I don't really know anyone here. Do you?"
"Yea," she says.
You give it one last shot. "Are you from around here?"
"Yea," she says.
Not a real talkative person.

Now there are different places you can go with this. In classic depressive fashion, you can decide that the problem is with you. You can think that this woman would talk to anybody else, but she senses something weird about you. You can prepare to flee.

Or you can go in a whole different direction.

You can decide that the woman doesn't want to talk, for whatever reason. Maybe she's in a bad mood. Maybe she has lousy social skills. You can realize that it has nothing to do with you. You don't know her. And she doesn't know you. You can decide further that you are not going to let her get you down. You then can walk on to another individual who also is standing alone and try again to start a conversation.

If you choose to go in the second direction, if you refuse to vilify yourself, you'll have just done something big. You'll have jumped a major hurdle in your efforts to overcome your fear and lessen your depression.

CONSIDER SPIRITUALITY

What is spirituality? Is it believing in God? Is it believing in an afterlife? Is it believing that energy forces draw us together? Is it questioning whether cells have memory? Is it questioning whether we have lived earlier lives? Is it asking whether we exist in parallel universes? Is it realizing that we are one with the universe?

Whether you are a religious person or not, it is important to realize that we are but a small part of whatever there is. So, when problems take over your world, go somewhere where you can be humbled by this realization. Give yourself up to the majesty, the complexity, the incredible nature of the world. Realize that you are lucky, incredibly lucky, to be here on earth.

I am not a religious person; I think I'm a spiritual person. I know there are things bigger than I. I believe that some things happen for a reason. I have had experiences in my life that have caused me to change course completely. I have met people whom I feel I have been meant to meet and I have met people whom I sense I have known before.

I'll tell you some stories. They are all true.

I wanted to build a room onto my house. I had talked to many contractors and all were too busy to take on a small project. I finally made arrangements with a distant cousin who was a contractor. Although he agreed to build the room for me, the completed room would not have all I wanted. When he had priced out my job, the cathedral ceiling I had hoped for exceeded my budget. I thought about contacting other contractors, but since getting any contractor to return my calls had proved so difficult, I decided to go with my cousin.

My cousin and I shook hands on the deal and I waited for him to begin. And waited. Calls to him got me nowhere. "I should be ready next week," he'd say. After nine months of holding on, I told him I was done waiting.

Now I was left with no one to build the room. I was very disappointed. I mentioned my dilemma to a few neighbors, but no one had any suggestions.

The next week, a stranger approached me when I was in the yard. "I'm your neighbor, Jay," he said. "I'm renting that house over there, renovating it, in fact, and I heard you needed a contractor."

I knew nothing about this man. Still, we got to talking about the project. I shared my ideas and he offered his. Two days later, Jay came over with a bid, one lower than my cousin's and including the cathedral ceiling.

I checked with my neighbors, but no one knew much about Jay. I asked Jay for his contractor's license. He stalled. "I'll get it to you later," he said. Later didn't come.

I confronted him. "O.K.," he said, "I don't have one."

Still, something told me to trust this guy. We agreed to work together.

Nine months later, my beautiful family room, complete with cathedral ceiling, was built. Jay and I had become friends. I had this weird feeling that I had a connection to Jay, that in some earlier time he was related to me, although I really don't believe in these things. Jay said he felt the connection too.

A week or two after completing my room, Jay stopped over.

"I have a present for you," he said.

Jay went out to his car and brought in a slightly worn, but beautiful, oriental rug.

"Here," he said. When I questioned him about the extravagance of the gift, he said he had nowhere to put the rug. I didn't believe him.

A few months later, the house Jay was renting and renovating was bought. The deal that he had made to stay in the house fell through. I never saw Jay again.

Isn't it odd that this man came out of nowhere, made my life more beautiful, and then disappeared?

Here's another story.

A few years after giving birth to my first child, I knew I wanted a second. But nature wasn't cooperating. After a period of time, my husband and I started looking into adoption. We were not candidates for traditional adoption agencies. We were past our early thirties, were of different religions and already had a biological child. These were all negatives for traditional adoption agencies.

After spending months looking into alternative routes to adoption, we began pursuing an independent adoption. This is an arrangement where prospective adoptive parents advertise for a birth mother looking to place her newborn for adoption (think the movie *Juno*).

We installed an 800 number into our home and started receiving phone calls. While all the calls were from nice women, the situations were not ones I was willing to consider.

Less than a month later, we received a call from a staff member at the adoption agency that had done our home study. Someone from a very well-known and traditional agency had been in touch with her. It appeared that one of that agency's contracts had fallen through. There had been a baby born, but the family who had agreed to take the newborn had backed out after learning that there was a seventy-five percent chance that the child would need heart surgery. Were we interested?

We had five days to decide.

I said we certainly wanted to consider it. Three hours later, we had what was known of the baby's medical information in hand.

With no appointment in place, I drove to our pediatrician's office and waited for our doctor to come out of an examining room. I quickly explained my dilemma. We needed someone to interpret the medical information. He instructed me to contact the head of pediatric cardiology at a well-known area hospital. He gave me the doctor's phone number.

I called the cardiologist, prepared to get his secretary or his answering machine, prepared to wait for days for a return call. Instead, the cardiologist answered the phone. (When does this ever happen?) I explained the situation. He offered to call the hospital in Indiana where our child had been born and talk to the attending doctor. (When does this ever happen?) He did and returned my call that afternoon. (When does this ever happen?) "It's routine surgery for us," he said. "I'd be comfortable with you going for it."

We agreed. We were going to adopt a baby girl.

If the story is not unusual enough, it gets more so. My family and I flew out to Indiana to meet our new daughter. Two weeks later, we were back in Boston, at the cardiologist's office. I wanted to talk about the surgery.

The cardiologist put our daughter through a variety of tests. Then he came out to talk to us. He was smiling. I figured it was because things were as he believed and the surgery would be, indeed, routine.

"Go home," he said.

I wasn't getting it.

"What?" I said.

"Go home," he said. "She's perfect. There's not a thing wrong with her."

"Wait a minute," I said. "That's impossible. She had a seventy-five percent chance of needing heart surgery. That's why we were considered to be her parents."

He continued to smile. "Go home," he said. "She's perfect. Consider it fate."

And one more story. A bittersweet one.

My nephew and niece had a friend. She was a wonderfully warm and loving human being, a defense attorney, a wife, and a mother. Years ago, Melanie got cancer. After a long, hard fight, she beat it. A year later, the cancer returned. I heard from my niece that she was very ill. Doctors were uncertain as to her prognosis. I often asked my niece about her. "Touch and go," she would say.

A few years ago, I saw her at a family function. Her hair was just growing back, having been lost to chemotherapy. She looked incredibly healthy and was beaming.

"You look great," I said. "How are you?"

"I'm wonderful," she said. "I feel better than I have ever felt."

Melanie went on to explain that her cancer had been a gift.

"I live so much more in the moment now," she said. "I'm so thankful for all my gifts." She pointed to her husband and her son. "For the gift of them. And all of you."

Melanie went on to explain that she had had to give up her practice, work that she had loved. She had fought a long, hard fight. She needed to preserve her strength and savor her family. She said it would be hard for her family financially but…

"The universe has a way of providing," she said.

Another year passed and I saw Melanie again. Her pain was obvious.

"How are you?" I asked.

"Not so good," she said. "The medication that was working so well stopped working. I'm on something new now. I don't know if it's working. The doctors say they don't know what else to do."

A little later she said, "There's a village in Peru that is known for its healers. If I get well enough, my son and I will go." Then she paused. "But it depends on what the universe wants for me. If I'm meant to live, I'll get well. But maybe I can do more good for the universe by dying. I'll have to see." Then she smiled and took my hand. "I have so many gifts. I'm so lucky."

So were all who knew her.

CHAPTER EIGHT

CHANGING YOUR BEHAVIOR

We have addressed your thoughts. By making use of a journal, you have learned more about how you think. By talking back to your thoughts, you have learned to see yourself more realistically. By realizing that you can change yourself, you have learned to see the half-built house of you as an awesome work-in-progress, as opposed to a project that will never be completed. By giving yourself true and complimentary statements, you have begun to acknowledge your strengths. By reality-testing your thoughts, you have learned that the world sees you more objectively and positively than you see yourself.

Now it is time to address your behaviors and get you ready to go out into the world.

ISOLATION

Twenty-first century America is an isolative place. Gone are the days when extended families lived together. Families are splintered. Biological dad lives on one side of the country, biological mom on the other. People marry two, three, four times. Stepbrothers and half-brothers live together until the family splits. One-time family members drift apart. Grandparents aren't cared for in the family home.

Jobs take us everywhere and drugs, alcohol, and divorce rip families apart.

Some of us, without family ties, make our own families. We find family in our coworkers, old high school or college friends, or teammates.

But many of the depressed people I know don't have jobs. Many haven't gone to college and their memories of high school are not worth remembering. They didn't play a sport. And they don't have the energy to reach out.

Their social networks are compromised. They feel isolated and alone.

To compensate, many of these people turn to television. Much too often, television becomes an all-day, everyday event.

I'll say it straight out. I've always been opposed to television. Rather maniacally opposed.

It's not the content that bothers me so much, although I think much of it is a waste of time. What bothers me is the process. Television is a passive activity. Unlike reading, it doesn't require us to spin words into pictures. Often it doesn't require that we think at all. From an evolutionary standpoint, television watching is detrimental to our progress. The less we humans think, the less we will be able to think.

And what is lost in the process of watching television?

When people spend their days watching television, they don't talk, read, dance, play guitar or soccer. If all-day television becomes a way of life, people forget that there is an exciting world out there. And television is a solitary affair. It takes the place of social connection, of friends.

That's why a key aspect of the mood-changing plan is to limit television to no more than three hours a day.

Often, people who are depressed are bored. They feel stuck. They think of all that they could have done with their lives, but haven't.

By limiting your television, you are opening up your world. You are giving yourself an invaluable opportunity to learn something new, add excitement to your life, and make yourself a more interesting person. In so doing, your confidence will increase and your depression will decrease.

What might you do with the time you had spent watching television? The choices are endless. You could study a foreign language, paint a picture, learn saxophone, race a car, compose music, start writing a novel, plant a garden, walk the beach, walk your dog, meet a potential partner, learn carpentry, sail a boat. In short, you can do anything you've ever wanted to do.

You will see that as part of the mood-changing calendar, you are asked to learn something new each week. This is important because the more you grow, the more you broaden your knowledge, the more intriguing you will find yourself. After a while, you will want to share the new you with others.

Limiting yourself to no more than three hours of television a day is essential.

HOW ABOUT THE COMPUTER?

When I was a kid, my friends and I talked on the phone or met out in the street with our hula hoops. If I had a question, I sat on the steps and waited to ask my mother. But the twenty-first-century world is a world of cyberspace. Now we text and email. If we have questions, we Google.

So what about the computer? Is it good for us? I think the key is moderation. While studies indicate that searching the web stimulates the brain and talking online is still connecting, we still need to go out and be with others. We still need to peer into another's big blues.

So what is the magic figure? How much computer use is too much? For the purposes of the mood-changing plan, keep computer use to two hours. Or replace your allotted television time with computer time.

Leave it like this. Use the computer as an add-on to a well-led life. Don't make it your life.

ADDRESS SUBSTANCE ABUSE

Many of the depressed people I know use alcohol. They do it to kick depression to the curb, to let loose, to numb out. And sometimes, for a night or two, it works. Shy people let their inhibitions fly. Serious people get funny. Quiet people get loud.

But what happens when people use alcohol on a continual basis? Does the fun continue? Of course, the answer is no. Long-term alcohol use leads only to a life measured from one drink to the next.

But alcohol is just one of many drugs.

O.K., here it goes. From my hip to yours. Most people like to let loose once in a while, have a drink with dinner, a few drinks at a party. And that's probably O.K. But consistent alcohol use is a cop-out, a short-term fix, Botox for the soul.

As for pot, I guess you need to decide. Just know that some people can't tolerate it, as it makes some anxious and others paranoid. And remember, too much of anything is too much.

There are deadlier drugs: crack, ecstasy, oxycodone, heroin, to name a few. In my opinion, playing with these drugs is like riding a Ferris wheel to the top, lifting the safety bar, and jumping out. Maybe you will live through your descent. Maybe you won't.

If you use drugs to cope, you will never learn to cope. And you will not grow.

The ultimate challenge in life is digging inside and becoming who you want to become on your own terms. Without crutches.

Taking on the challenge of becoming you is the ultimate life adventure. It is how you beat depression.

For the purposes of the mood-changing plan, I am asking you to refrain from substance abuse.

You know what this means.

START GOING OUT

Studies find that people who are connected to others are happy.

Limiting your television time is a gift. It is giving you hours in the day that you didn't have before. It's giving you time to connect with others.

But what constitutes connection?

One of my very isolated clients goes out a few times a week. She goes to a coffee shop where she knows no one, buys a donut, and sits by herself. Week after week she goes to this coffee shop, often seeing the same people. Sometimes, she and another woman acknowledge each other with a greeting, but they do not engage in conversation. My client remains depressed.

"How about talking to this woman?" I ask.

"I don't know her," she says.

"You could," I say.

"I don't know," my client says.

"What's the worst that could happen?" I ask.

"Maybe she won't want to talk to me," she says.

"Maybe she will," I say.

As part of your mood-changing plan, I am asking that you go somewhere where there are others, preferably others whom you know or with whom you have things in common, and initiate at least two conversations.

Spend at least two hours a week on this work. If it is easier for you to spread this time out, do so. But don't cut this work short. The point of these excursions is to give you an opportunity to interact with others and, ultimately, make friends. When friends enter your life, isolation exits.

Friends are so important. They give you a reason to get up, go to lunch, go fishing, or play cards. They cause you to smile, laugh, goof off. If you have friends, make the time to meet with them. If your friends isolate even more than you, take the initiative and arrange get-togethers. If you have lost the friends who were once in your life, work at making new ones. Ask yourself where you can find people who might share your interests. Guys with Harleys like to talk sidecars and weekend rides. Mountain climbers like to talk tall peaks. Readers like to talk books, film buffs, films. Having things in common makes conversations a whole lot easier.

So where can you find people with whom you have things in common? The answer is simple. Go where they are. If you are a biker looking to talk bikes, join a local motorcycle group. Or call your local Harley dealer and find out if there are any events coming up. If you are a bicycler, join a bike club. If you are a reader, join a book club. If you have a two-year-old, join a play group. If exercise is your thing, take a class at the YMCA. If church is a big part of your life, take part in your church's social activities. If you struggle with alcoholism, go to AA. If depression is your number one concern, join a depression support group.

If you are more of a generalist and don't have an interest which consumes you, you may want to opt for meeting people at more common gathering spots. Lots of my clients meet people at Dunkin' Donuts. The sixty-five-year-old daughter of my neighbor met the new guy in her life at McDonald's. From what I hear, people are pretty receptive to those who smile.

Here are some more ideas for places to connect: Starbucks; dinner at a restaurant, seated at the bar; the dog park; the pet store; the park; any place where people walk their dogs; dog training classes; the beach; ice cream stands; the local fishing dock; kids' sporting activities; the book store; the library; art classes; art galleries; yoga classes; swing or country dance classes; Home Depot's how-to workshops; adult education classes; block parties, and other community events.

My list is just that—mine. Now you need to make yours.

If you don't like the idea of going out alone, take a buddy. If a friend invites you to go somewhere with her, go. But remember, this is your work. It is your job to start conversations with people. If your friend is the one doing the talking, it doesn't count.

Some depressed people are shy. A lot of depressed people lack self-confidence. The thought of interacting with anyone is scary. When forced to talk to near-strangers, they panic. I understand. When I get nervous, my mouth gets dry, my lips tremble, and my feet get stuck, like the floor has glue on it. Then I remember that I've been told that I walk like a camel and all is lost.

What many shy, depressed people don't realize is that making conversation is a learned art. We all get better with practice.

So what are the rules of conversation?

Make neutral comments. Ask questions for which there are neither right nor wrong answers. Give people the opportunity to talk about themselves. Be generous with your compliments.

Let's try an example. Suppose it's a spring afternoon and you are at your daughter's soccer game, standing next to someone you don't know.

Using the "make neutral comments" approach, you might start a conversation like this: "Good thing spring's here, huh? We sure paid the price with the weather this winter," or "My daughter's new to soccer this year, but she's having a good time. Seems like a good team."

Here's another example, employing all the techniques.

Suppose you are out walking your lab and you come upon someone else with a dog. Start with something neutral. "Your dog's cute. What kind is he?" No matter what he answers, follow up. If he says, "He's a border collie," you might say something like, "Oh, they're supposed to be so smart." If you don't know anything about the breed, ask a question or make a comment. "Are they hunting dogs?" or "Have you had him since he was a puppy?" or "He really seems to listen to you."

And yet another example.

Suppose you are at a party and don't know a soul. You are uncomfortable standing alone. You wish someone would talk to you. You wish you were home in your sweat pants. Then, you remember—you need to take the initiative. You need to start a conversation. So what do you do?

Find someone standing alone and begin with a neutral comment. "This house is so cool," or "The food here looks so awesome. What I wouldn't give to have my own chef." Or, "I just realized I'm missing my favorite TV show. Good thing I'm taping it."

In general, sports are good topics, but sports fanatics are… fanatical. Don't sing the praises of the Yankees if you are in Red Sox country. Politics are equally dicey. There are zealots on every side. Make your comments general unless you want to get into a brawl. While standing in line at a grocery store for a half-pound of ham, I almost got into a hair pull over Iraq. And unless you want out-and-out war, keep your religious beliefs to yourself.

Becoming a good conversationalist takes practice. Use every opportunity to work on your skills. And remember, most people are more concerned with how they look and sound than with how you look or sound. And people are just people. Most snore and have rolls of fat somewhere.

One other suggestion. Before going out, read the paper or watch the news. If you know what is going on in the world, you will be more comfortable holding your own.

In asking you to go out, I am asking you to go somewhere and connect with others. Start conversations. If the person you approach responds, great. Engage in a conversation. Who knows? A friendship might ensue. If the person blows you off, don't take it personally. Pride yourself on the fact that you are honing your techniques. The more you develop your conversational skills, the better you will feel about yourself.

Go different places. Try your hand with different people. Remember, people are not doing you a favor talking to you. You have something to offer.

I know this is scary. But connecting with others and making friends will do much to conquer your depression.

This is hard work. Reward yourself after each time you go out.

VOLUNTEERING

Depression skews our vision. It's too much time turned inward. After a while, our problems are the only problems we see. Our pain becomes the definition of pain. We forget there is a world out there.

Volunteering helps get us out of ourselves. It puts us in touch with the needs of others, needs that are often bigger than ours. Volunteering lets us make a difference in other people's lives. By helping others, we realize we matter.

Specifically, I am asking that you volunteer your time at least once a week for a minimum of two hours.

Where you volunteer is up to you. But make your choice meaningful. If you love kids, consider becoming a Big Sister or volunteering at a children's hospital. If the isolation and warehousing of our elders upsets you, consider volunteering at a nursing home or becoming an ombudsman and fighting for the rights of the elderly. If you are disturbed by the fact that men, women, and children are sleeping in the cold and eating out of dumpsters, consider volunteering at a homeless shelter, soup kitchen, or food bank. If you love animals and are bothered by the thought of all those without homes, consider volunteering at a no-kill animal shelter or rescue league.

To find volunteer opportunities, call around. Some places, such as hospitals, have volunteer departments. If the organization you are calling does not, ask to speak with the person in charge. Sometimes, it takes more than one phone call. Be persistent and know that you have something to offer.

EXERCISE

Exercise is a key part of your mood-changing plan. You are being asked to exercise a minimum of two times per week for at least a half hour a time. One of these times needs to be with other people. For your exercise with others, consider taking an aerobics class at the YMCA, a yoga class at the community center, a kick-boxing class… Also, in addition to this exercise, I'm asking you to take two walks per week, alone, with your dog, or with a friend.

The reason for exercising is obvious. Studies find that people who exercise regularly experience lower rates of depression.

When you exercise, your body releases chemicals called endorphins. Endorphins interact with receptors in your brain and trigger feelings of well-being.

Exercise has other payoffs too. Many depressed people are overweight. Some of the medications they have taken to help themselves have caused them to put on weight. And too often they have used food for comfort.

The more exercise you do, the more weight you'll lose and the more toned you'll be. This, of course, will lead people to compliment you on how good you look, which will make you feel better. And feeling better will translate into being less depressed. Yes, exercise tones the body, takes off weight, releases feel-good chemicals in the brain, and sets the stage for receiving a slew of compliments. It's a win, win, win, win situation.

Exercise also allows you to get out of the house, to breathe the air. And it can be social. There are walking and biking clubs, aerobics and dance classes, rock climbing events... There are Mommy and Me classes for new moms and ballroom dancing for seniors. There are basketball leagues for guys just out of college and for guys in their fifties.

Be consistent with your exercise. Set a particular hour. Determine a specific amount of time. Take a class with someone else. Tell everyone you know. You may not want to exercise. Do it anyway. It is a requirement of the plan and you will feel better afterward.

CHANGE YOUR DIET

Remember when mom told you that you are what you eat. Well... If you eat red meat for breakfast, lunch, and dinner; if pasta and other carbohydrates are your definition of food; if white is the only color choice in your diet; if you go from one fast-food place to another; if you eat dessert first; if fish and berries are a once a year thing, you need to alter your diet.

Food is meant to provide us with nutrients and give energy to our days. It is also meant to keep our systems and our moods in balance. But much of the food we eat today is nutritionally empty. The wrong food weighs us down or bloats us up like so many buoys in the harbor. It fosters depression, creates difficulties with our concentration, and causes long-term health problems.

Our diets have a tremendous influence on our brain's behavior. What we eat significantly impacts how well our neurotransmitters function (neurotransmitters or brain chemicals such as serotonin, dopamine, and norepinephrine regulate behavior and are closely linked with mood). When we have too much or too little of these brain chemicals or when these chemicals are out of balance, emotional disturbances can occur. Enough protein and complex carbohydrate consumption and absorption, as well as ample intake of fatty acids, vitamin B, folate, magnesium, and other nutrients are necessary for maintaining the building blocks required to synthesize neurotransmitters.

So what does all this mean?

Eating a Mediterranean diet, or one similar, with emphasis on vegetables, fruits, nuts, seeds, whole grains, legumes, fish, and olive oil is believed to go a long way toward warding off depression. The reason? These foods offer us the essential vitamins and nutrients necessary for truly healthy living.

Let's look at where support for a Mediterranean diet comes from. A well-publicized 2006 study by A. Sanchez-Villegas, P. Henriquez, M. Bes-Rastrollo, and J. Doreste from the University of Las Palmas de Gran Canaria, Spain, focused on whether the adherence to a Mediterranean diet, which is high in Omega-3 and B vitamins, including folic acid, could be protective against depression. As part of the study, data from almost ten thousand participants was analyzed. The results were interesting.

There were no statistically significant associations between B-6 vitamin intake and depression. Less than sufficient folate intake appears associated with depression, particularly among men, and especially among smokers. Less than sufficient B-12 intake was associated with depression among women, particularly among smokers, and those women who were physically active.

Ample fatty acid intake appears associated with decreased depression in women.

The ultimate conclusion?

A Mediterranean diet with its ample supply of B vitamins and nutrients can be protective against depression. Put another way, a diet of fruit, vegetables, nuts, seeds, legumes, whole grains, fish, and olive oil will go a long way toward making your brain function optimally. An everyday diet of meat, dairy, chips, and chocolate cake and your moods will be a crap shoot.

Fish, with or without the Mediterranean diet, is another hot topic when it comes to depression.

In 1996, The Journal of the American Medical Association published a study comparing rates of depression across ten nations. In Taiwan, one to two percent of adults reported experiencing depression. In Beirut, almost twenty percent reported experiencing depression. Why the difference? A study published in The Lancet in 1998 offered an answer: the higher the fish consumption among populations, the lower the rates of depression. Another study noted that in Japan and Taiwan, where there is higher fish consumption (and thus higher consumption of Omega-3) than in North America, the rates of depression are ten times lower than in North America.

The working ingredient of fish oil is Omega-3, found in plants such as flaxseed, pumpkin seed, and walnuts. Dr. Joseph Hibbeln, of the National Institute of Health, who authored the fish-consumption studies said, "In the last century, [Western] diets have radically changed and we eat grossly fewer Omega-3 fatty acids now. We also know that rates of depression have radically increased by perhaps a hundred-fold."

In a New York Times article, Dr. Hibbeln reported that "Depression is sixty times higher in New Zealand than in Japan. In New Zealand, the average consumption of seafood is 40 pounds per year compared to Japan, where a person consumes nearly 150 pounds of seafood a year." He also noted that Omega-3 appears to be critical to the growth and maintenance of brain cells, particularly cell membranes. When Omega-3 is not available, the body relies on Omega-6, which produces cell membranes less able to cope with neurotransmitter traffic.

In his 2001 book *The Omega-3 Connection*, Dr. Andrew Stoll, then Director of the Psychopharmacology Research Laboratory at McLean Hospital in Belmont, Massachusetts, explained how food and depression are related. In Paleolithic times, man's diet consisted primarily of fruits, vegetables, nuts, seeds, fish, and wild game. It was a diet high in essential Omega-3 fatty acids. It was the diet on which modern man's brain evolved and, per Dr. Stoll, the diet on which the twenty-first-century brain is meant to be nourished.

Like others have, Dr. Stoll pointed out that the brain does not function optimally without adequate amounts of Omega-3 and that deficiencies in Omega-3 are linked to depression. As Dr. Stoll noted, the body cannot make Omega-3 on its own, so it must obtain these fatty acids through diet or supplements. It is known that fatty fish, such as salmon, mackerel, herring, lake trout, sardines, and albacore tuna, as well as seeds and nuts, are great sources of Omega-3.

Unfortunately, it is known that North Americans do not consume sufficient fatty fish, seeds, or nuts. So what's a good North American to do? Either eat more fish or take an Omega-3 supplement. Some studies also have indicated that Omega-3 supplements, when taken in addition to antidepressants, can make antidepressants more effective.

What about other vitamins and supplements?

Folic acid, also called folate, is a B vitamin that often is lacking in people who are depressed. Vitamin B-6 is necessary for the adequate production of mood-enhancing neurotransmitters, while B-12 helps with moods and irritability. A deficiency in B-1 can cause problems with fatigue and irritability. Vitamin D is another important supplement, particularly for those suffering from Seasonal Affective Disorder. And ample magnesium is necessary to keep depression at bay.

Lots of information and lots of choices. So what do you do?

My opinion is this: Eat a Mediterranean diet or one similar. Try to have fish twice a week. Drink lots of water. Avoid sugar, alcohol, soda, processed and refined foods, and junk food as they are lousy for your body and your moods. Choose olive oil over vegetable oil or butter. Include at least five servings of vegetables and fruits daily. Choose whole grains over white bread and white rice. Whenever possible, choose fresh food over frozen. Take supplements unless your diet is consistently healthy.

To help determine which fruits and vegetables to eat, nature has provided a color code. Dark and bright are the tickets. So, pretend you are a brown bear and go for the goodies that stand out.

Your body is the only one you've got. Nurture it.

SLEEP IS HUGE

Sleep problems and depression are related.

Many depressed people have trouble falling asleep, staying asleep, or sleeping at all. Still others sleep too much. Which comes first? Do sleep problems cause depression? Or does depression cause sleep problems? The answer is unclear.

Insomnia is very common among those who are depressed. Studies note that individuals with insomnia have a much greater risk (some studies say ten times greater) of developing depression than those who sleep well. In the category of kids and teens eleven to seventeen, those who report feeling significantly depressed also report sleep difficulties. Among adolescents and adults, those with sleep problems and depression tend to have more significant depression than those who sleep well.

Sleep problems and depression may share biological roots and often respond to the same treatment. Translated, this means that sleep problems and depression both may resolve with the use of an antidepressant. However, if you find that your mood improves with an antidepressant, but your sleep problems do not, discuss this with your doctor. There may be an underlying sleep disorder that requires different treatment.

What tips help ensure a good night's sleep?

Try to go to bed at the same time each night. Try to awaken around the same time each morning. Our bodies get used to a sleep cycle.

If you find yourself sleeping during the day, stop. Unless you have a physical condition that requires you to nap, your nighttime sleep should be sufficient. Many people sleep during the day because they find coping with life too difficult. Use the exercises in this book to fill and invigorate your day.

Try taking a shower or bath before going to bed. Warm water is soothing. If possible, give yourself several hours to relax in bed before you need to sleep. If you find yourself thinking too much, write your thoughts on a note pad and leave the pad by your bedside. This way you know your thoughts will be there in the morning and you won't stay up worrying about forgetting them. Read or listen to a relaxation tape. Avoid television before bed as it is too stimulating. Avoid soda or coffee at night.

If these techniques don't work, talk to your doctor. She may prescribe a medication.

Sleeping is your time to recharge. Make it a priority.

ADD LIGHT

Our bodies are affected by the amount of light to which we are exposed. Getting plenty of natural sunshine, with its wavelengths of infrared to ultraviolet light, is known to help fight depression. But a lot of us don't live in places where sunshine is a given the majority of the year. What effect does this have?

Just like sunny days make most of us happy, too many gray days make many of us sad. But people with Seasonal Affective Disorder have even stronger responses to seasonal changes in light. Typically, people with this disorder begin to feel their moods plummet in fall as darkness takes up more of the day. Then in spring, when the days grow longer, their moods improve. The reason for this is biological. Circadian rhythms are regulated by the body's internal clock and by exposure to sunshine. When the days get shorter in fall, circadian rhythms become desynchronized. Depression often results. In spring, as the days get longer, depression decreases.

Those with Seasonal Affective Disorder often benefit from bright light therapy. This therapy employs full-spectrum light (housed in a light box) that simulates natural daylight. Sitting two to three feet in front of a light box, for one half to two hours a day (the time depends on the intensity of the light), preferably in mornings, helps most people with Seasonal Affective Disorder. It is not necessary to stare into the light. People can do whatever it is they wish while sitting in close proximity to the light box. It is suggested that people with Seasonal Affective Disorder begin this treatment in autumn when the days begin to shorten. Many people using bright light therapy see dramatic improvements within a few weeks.

Bright light therapy also has been shown to work for other disorders. Several studies have demonstrated that three weeks of bright light therapy improved symptoms of depression and sleep problems in over fifty percent of older adults.

It appears that bright light therapy optimizes levels of serotonin, a neurotransmitter associated with depression, in much the same way as antidepressants do.

Bright light therapy may provide an alternative for those who cannot tolerate treatment with antidepressants.

Does exposure to bright light therapy always help? The answer is no. People with Bipolar Disorder may be catapulted into mania by exposure to too much light.

Artificial dawn-dusk simulators also seem to help with depression. Our internal body clocks are set by the amount of light and darkness to which we are exposed. During the winter months, we are attempting to awaken while our bodies, still producing the sleep hormone melatonin, are telling us it is nighttime and time to sleep. By initiating sunrise with an artificial dawn-dusk simulator, we are stopping the production of melatonin and allowing our bodies to awaken more naturally. As we have seen, improving our ability to sleep helps fight depression.

Sleeping without any light at night also appears to keep depression at bay. Research conducted at Ohio State University showed that female Siberian hamsters exposed to dim light (5 lux, roughly the amount of light emitted from a television in a darkened room) nightly for eight weeks experienced significant physical changes in the hippocampus, provoking depressive-like behaviors. Hamsters who spent the night in complete darkness exhibited fewer depressive behaviors.

Researchers believe that sleeping in darkness at night, without so much as the light of a television, is beneficial for mood.

In short, getting as much natural light as possible, even in winter; using a light box if necessary; and sleeping in darkness will help with depression. So, too, will allowing as much light as possible into your home during winter months. Choosing curtains that let in light are a better choice than curtains that block out the sun. Keeping your curtains or shades up during the day in winter is even better.

Remember, when the worst of winter is here, spring is creeping right behind.

ADD COLOR

Why do colors have such an effect on our moods?

Color is a form of visible light. We know the impact sunlight has on our moods, so why should we expect any less from color?

But why do particular colors impact our moods so differently? Why do people who walk through fields of sunflowers feel happy? Why are so many bedrooms painted blue? Why are the colors red, yellow, and orange used so frequently in restaurants?

According to Dr. Morton Walker, author of *The Power of Color*, color affects both our physical and emotional well-being. The color blue makes us feel tranquil, while green helps us heal. Orange grabs our attention, red energizes and sparks our passions, and yellow makes us happy. And white, the color we see when all colors come together, makes us feel pure, innocent, and at peace.

Some of my clients complain about their homes being drab. Often, I suggest they paint something: a piece of furniture, a wall, a room, the whole house. Adding color changes everything. And color often adds the spark that's needed. This is particularly true if they are colors you love.

For me, these colors are red and yellow. For whatever reasons, walls painted these colors make me hungry. If there is any stonework near the red and yellow walls, I find myself famished and in search of cheese and hearty breads.

Choose colors you love. Be daring; it's only paint. When you're done painting, sit back and appreciate it. If it's a piece of furniture you've painted, put it in a central spot. Put your feet on it. Enjoy.

FOLLOW YOUR NOSE

Aromatherapy is a centuries-old tradition that pays homage to the world's flora, the treks of the bees, and man's determination to find ways to honor the gods, temper or embolden the emotions, and heal both body and soul. It is a tradition that utilizes aromatic essences (referred to as extracts or oils) from plants, flowers, and fruits. Different oils have different properties, thus produce different effects. Lavender is known to calm and encourage sleep, rose and geranium to soothe depression, orange to energize, ylang-ylang and rosemary to temper anger.

There are many ways to enjoy aromatherapy.

If you have a passion for things French (as I do), you will sprinkle lavender on your pillows (underneath your cases) and dream of sunflowers and stone walls. Those who survive nasty New England snowstorms only by counting the hours until a warm soak in a tub, will want to look into bath mixtures. I am told that a combination of honey, lavender, basil, and geranium is very nice. Room diffusers are a way for those with roommates to share the joy. Massage oils are popular. Scented candles are romantic. Some herbs can be added to teas, others to exotic and not so exotic dishes. The list goes on.

If aromatherapy sounds like a sweet way to feel better, do a little research. Before long, you and your personal space will smell so good you will forget to feel bad.

WORK WITH A THERAPIST

The mood-changing activities described in this book can be done without the help of a therapist. Yet, therapy is very helpful and I suggest you add it to your plan.

Why?

Often, depression has its roots in criticism or abuse. Reaching a depression-free zone in life can be a potholed road. Working with a therapist is like getting the county workers to fill in the holes so driving goes a lot smoother.

All children depend on their caretakers for survival. Many kids, who have been overly criticized or abused, learn to stuff what they feel. They learn to keep secrets. Having no outlet for their pain and fury, they turn these things inward.

Skilled therapists can help people come into their own. They help those who don't believe in themselves, believe. They help those who have been abused realize they didn't deserve the abuse they suffered. They help them see they were not to blame. So often, abuse victims hate themselves, believing they were somehow complicit in the behaviors they found despicable.

With enough work, people who have suffered at the hands of others can learn to let go of their rage. They learn to find freedom from their torment. They learn that while they may never forget and may never forgive, they can move on. They can resume life among the living.

WHAT KIND OF THERAPIES DO PEOPLE NEED?

There are different schools of therapy, each with their own techniques. However, most therapists are not wed to one school of thought, but rather, use a variety of different approaches. The goal of most therapy is to help clients change those behaviors that are no longer healthy.

Throughout this book, I have talked about a specific type of therapy, known as Cognitive or Cognitive Behavior Therapy. Cognitive therapy is based on the premise that thoughts precede feelings and that what we think determines how we feel. If our thoughts tell us what jerks we are, we feel lousy. If our thoughts tell us how awesome we are, we feel great. Cognitive therapy teaches us to question our distorted thoughts. Behavior therapy has as its focus behaviors needing change. It is based on the work of B.F. Skinner and Joseph Wolpe. Skinner introduced a technique called Operant Conditioning. The premise behind operant conditioning is that individuals choose behaviors based on past or present consequences. Wolpe demonstrated that people can be treated for phobias by increasingly tolerating the stimuli that provokes their anxieties. Cognitive Behavior Therapy combines both cognitive and behavioral theory. It helps us look at our distorted thoughts and change the behaviors that result from them.

Psychodynamic therapy attempts to help clients understand the origins of their dysfunctional behaviors. Therapists from this school of thought believe that if individuals understand the roots of their problems, they will be better able to change their behaviors.

If I were to define myself, I would say I am a cognitive behavioral therapist who is eclectic. Eclectic means using a variety of approaches. I believe most other therapists would say they are eclectic as well.

HOW DO YOU FIND A GOOD THERAPIST?

I do not believe all therapists are created equal any more than I believe that all artists or all athletes are created equal.

So how do you find a good therapist?

Start by asking people you know and respect. Recommendations are invaluable. If you ask your primary care doctor, ask if she has patients who have spoken highly of a particular therapist. If you have a psychiatrist, ask if she has a recommendation. If she gives you a name, ask her what her clients say about the therapist. Look up the websites for reputable psychiatric hospitals and see if they list therapists who are affiliated with them. Look on your medical insurance's website and see if there are write-ups of the therapists they mention. If you have a specific disorder such as depression or Obsessive Compulsive Disorder, find a website that specializes in this disorder and read about the therapists who are mentioned.

Speak with the therapist on the phone before you meet her. How does she sound? Are you comfortable talking with her? Then, meet her. Do you feel good about her? Do you feel you can be open with her? Does she seem nonjudgmental? Go with your gut. If you don't like her, find another. So much of the therapeutic process is about the relationship. My personal opinion is this: No matter how big your struggle, you always should leave a session feeling better than when you arrived.

TAP INTO YOUR CREATIVITY

When I'm bored, I know something is wrong. Boredom is a signal that I'm trying to run from my emotions.

If I don't do something quickly, sadness comes from around the corner of my boredom and tackles me.

Like most good women, I find shopping a quick fix. But shopping is expensive. So sometimes, instead of shopping, I go inside myself and tap into my creativity.

I love color, particularly reds and yellows, and stone. So when I'm bored, I come up with a project. I paint a wall, flowers on the treads of the stairs, vines on a hutch. Or I gather stones and try to make a walkway in the garden. I'm not a good painter and I am not a mason. But my projects are just that—my projects.

As part of your mood-changing plan, I've asked you to try something new each week. At least once a month, make that something new come from within you. Is music your thing? Try playing an instrument. Learn the guitar or piano or sax. Play the drums. If you can't afford lessons, turn to the internet. There's a YouTube video for everything.

Maybe you have always wanted to write. Don't say you can't write. We all have stories inside. Forget everything you learned in English class. A good writer breaks the rules. Your spin makes your work unique.

Do you want to build a boat? Design clothes? Write songs?

Do whatever it is you've always wanted to do.

When you let your creative genie loose, you are relying on yourself to shake up your world.

So go for it. Let others get a peek at your soul. Wow yourself and anyone else who's around.

SPEND TIME WITH ANIMALS

Animals are a gift. They ask for so little and give so much. It takes so little to make them happy. They are so loyal. And the love they give you is profound. If you have a dog or cat, spend time with him. Forget that you are depressed and don't want to do anything. Think of him. Think of all he gives you.

One of my clients has polio. It is hard for her to get around and she is always in pain. The cold wreaks havoc on her body. Life has been tough for her. She has little contact with her family and lives on disability. She runs out of money monthly.

Yet, she has a dog to whom she is devoted. Every day, in good weather or bad, she walks her dog. They walk for blocks, she with her brace. After a new snow, she takes her dog to the park and laughs as her pup leaps into the snow banks. Seeing her dog happy makes her happy.

Walking her dog has helped her have a social life. When she and her pup walk, she meets others who are out walking their dogs. Recently, my client thought she might have to move. When she shared this information with a casual neighbor, the neighbor expressed her dismay. "Seeing you two together makes me smile," said the neighbor. "I hope you don't move. It wouldn't be the same around here."

Another client with whom I worked had nothing. No family, no friends, no job, and for the third and fourth week of each month, no money. She smoked cigarettes, drank beer, and ate turkey dogs and rice. Then she was given a cat. She named him Riley. Riley was very shy, but my client was patient and spent time with him. Eventually, Riley came out to play. When I would meet my client for a session, she would talk about Riley. "He's so sweet," she would say. He needed her. One of the last times I saw this client, she had cut herself back to four cigarettes a day so she could afford tuna for Riley. "He deserves it," she said. "He makes me so happy."

It doesn't have to be a dog or cat to make you happy. It can be a hamster. Or a ferret. One of my clients had two ferrets. They made her laugh.

Go for a walk with your dog, sit on the couch with your cat, play with your hamster, watch your ferret sleep. Tell him how good he is. It will do great things for both of you.

If you don't have an animal, and feel that you cannot afford to get one, stop on your walks to say hello to the dogs you see. Or consider volunteering at an animal shelter.

CHAPTER NINE

CHOOSING FROM THE B LIST

Chances are you did a whole lot more when you weren't depressed. Do you remember what you did? Did you have more fun?

Most depressed people don't do a whole lot with their time. They certainly don't do as much as they used to do. They sleep too much. They watch too much television.

When I ask my clients why they don't do more, they say they are depressed. They say they have no motivation. But here's the catch. Depressed people don't feel like doing much. But the less they do, the more depressed they become.

My father used to say that the best way to beat depression was to stay busy and eat bran. I don't know about the bran part, but he was right about the busy.

Depressed or not, you have to keep going.

There's an exercise therapists use to challenge clients' lack of motivation. Clients are asked to rate their motivation on a scale of 0 to 10 before engaging in activities and their enjoyment of the activities after.

The results? You guessed it.

People who are depressed don't want to do anything. The thought of engaging in any activity makes them pull those scratchy, wool covers that much higher over their heads. But after doing the activity, clients realize, dare I say it, that they just may have enjoyed themselves.

Waiting for motivation is a huge mistake. It's like waiting for the ice cream truck to crawl down one of Boston's North End streets in the middle of February.

There is a varied and textured life out there. By refusing to hold out for motivation in their willingness to act, clients rediscover the joy of living.

Once a week you are being asked to choose an activity from the "B List" and spend an hour and a half on it. The activities on the "B List" are unlike your "Learn Something New" activities. Activities on the "B List" are things you may have done in the past when the world still excited you, when you had things to talk about, when life was about living. Others on the list are activities that would have been interesting, had you ever gotten around to them. Well, the time has come.

THE B LIST

READ THE NEWSPAPER

Depressed people know their inner worlds. They know what they think, what they feel, and every little thing that is wrong with them. But what they forget is that there is a very big world out there.

How long has it been since you have paid attention to that world?

Whose governments have been toppled?

What natural disasters has the world survived?

Whose lost dogs have crossed three state lines to find their owners?

What acts of bravery have gone unheralded?

Knowing what's going on in the world connects us to others. It helps us realize that all the world's citizens share a common humanity.

On a more practical basis, it gives us things to talk about and makes us more interesting people.

So read a newspaper.

Buying a daily newspaper can be expensive. But newspapers can be read for free at local libraries and at most Dunkin' Donuts. And there's always the online news.

So go. Find out what's happening out there in the world.

WATCH THE NEWS

Same as "Read the Newspaper," but watching television does the visuals for you. Everybody has their favorite news channel, but I like CBS.

TURN ON MUSIC

Some people find music invigorating. Others find it relaxing. And everybody has a favorite thing.

Some are into rock, others are into jazz or blues, others into classical. As for me—it's country or nothing. And I'm serious about the nothing. Sometimes I just like to listen to the wind.

But whatever you like, there's music out there for you. Janis Joplin going wild, Toby Keith going crazy, Beethoven being Beethoven, waves lapping the shore. Turn on your radio or plug in your iPod, close your eyes, and get carried away.

PLAY CARDS

My grandfather taught me that a good woman knows how to play a good game of gin rummy and shuffle a mean deck of cards. He also taught me that red traffic lights are not nearly as important as the police make them out to be.

My grandfather was a pharmacist. He was happily married. But even after his wife died, my grandfather went on to live a long and enjoyable life. Gin rummy had much to do with this.

My grandfather was a member of the Elks. During his working years and after, he would go to the Elks daily to play gin rummy. He didn't care who he played and he didn't play for big stakes, just a quarter a game. He had fun whether he won or lost, although I think he was known for winning.

Because of his rummy games, he was invited on yearly, free jaunts to Vegas. He thought this was so funny. "I play for a quarter a game," he'd say. "What do they want with me?" But he loved going. He always took two hundred dollars on these trips. "Won't spend a penny more," he'd say. "Unless I win." And he didn't.

In his late eighties, my grandfather lived in a motel in the heart of Miami, with many other elderly people. He chose this motel because it was within walking distance of the Elks. He didn't have much money, but he looked forward to his days and his games of gin rummy. He lamented the fact that so many of his rummy partners had died off. "I make plans for a game today and tomorrow the guy's not there because he's dead. It's sad," he'd say. Still, he'd walk to the Elks and find someone with whom he could play.

My grandfather lived a good life. He remained independent. He looked forward to his days. Gin rummy was his passion and his reason to get up.

If you have a passion and it doesn't hurt anyone, keep it as part of your life.

WATCH MONDAY NIGHT FOOTBALL

Football has its adoring fans, both young and old, and its honored celebrations-Monday Night Football and Super Bowl Sunday.

Those who live for football feel it in their blood. They wear the shirts and know the stats.

They live each play as if they were doing the playing. They have their own fantasy teams. Their football greats are heroes who rival the likes of Teddy Roosevelt.

One of my clients is seventy-six years old. He is depressed and worried about his memory. He doesn't look forward to much. He goes to bed by seven-thirty p.m. and wakes up tired. But on nights when football is being played, he stays up until the game is over. He remembers when he played football in high school and how exhilarating it felt. The day after each game his eyes sparkle as he tells anyone who will listen all the details of his favorite plays.

WRITE IN A JOURNAL

I've already talked about this, but journals are wonderful tools. What better way to figure out what you're thinking than to think aloud on paper. So that you can be really honest, keep your journal private. Buy a journal with a key. Remember, you don't owe it to anyone to share your thoughts.

If having a journal with a key is impossible or if you think that those around you will refuse to honor your privacy, going so far as to pry your journal's lock, consider using a dry erase board. Ponder your thoughts, write them down, and wipe clean.

I've already said it, but I'll say it again. Don't wait for inspiration. Besides, what people call inspiration is ninety-five percent hard work. Set a daily time to write and stick to this time.

DANCE

It seems that we humans have been dancing forever. Since the earliest human civilizations, dance has given voice to our emotions and our passions.

Dance frees us to speak wordlessly. Of chaos, loss, hope, desire, want, and dreams.

So turn on the country music, the salsa, the rock-and-roll, the jazz, the blues, the hip-hop. Move to what you feel. Seduce. Leap like a gazelle. Soar like a bird.

CALL A GOOD FRIEND

A good friend is someone who cares, who goes out of her way for you, who doesn't judge. If you are lucky enough to have one, call her. Remember to ask how she's doing too. No matter how good a friend she is, she still wants to know that you care about her.

BRING DINNER TO A FRIEND

A few years ago, to celebrate my birthday, a friend came over with a homemade dinner of curried shrimp. She also brought a homemade chocolate dessert. I remember thinking how wonderful this was. This friend and I often exchanged presents on our birthdays, but this present was special. She knew how much I loved curried shrimp. And desserts, particularly chocolate... well, I've always lived by the motto: "Life's short. Eat dessert first."

While sweet, it's easy to buy someone a present. But to make something from scratch, to plan out a menu and sweat in front of a stove, this says something. To me it said, "You're special enough for me to put in the effort."

JOIN FACEBOOK AND RECONNECT

I thought Facebook was just for kids until I read a few articles saying adults were using it too. O.K., I thought, why not? I had lost contact with so many people from my past. Some of them were people I had loved a lot.

Still, I didn't expect much.

On I went. Instructions on Facebook said you could look up people by name. I wondered what the odds were of finding my old friends this way. After all, there are a lot of John Smiths and a few Cathy Goldsteins. But what the hey, I figured. I'd give it a try. Continuing to read, I learned that you could cross-reference people by name and the high school or college they had attended and their years of attendance. It seemed as if the odds were getting better.

My first night on Facebook, I found a man who had been much like a brother to me when I was in my twenties, and a woman who had been my best friend when I lived in Colorado. I also had a lead on a guy with whom I had crossed the country when I was freshman in college. He and I had driven a thousand miles to see a rock concert, only to fall asleep on top of his van and miss all but the concert's clean-up crew.

Although I couldn't see their profiles that first night, I sent a message to each.

By the next day, two of the three friends I had contacted had responded. They, too, were happy we had found each other.

In just a few months on Facebook. I found and connected with everyone for whom I looked. I can't tell you how much fun it's been and how it feels as if I had gone home for Thanksgiving and everyone I ever loved was there.

MAKE A NEW FRIEND

Remember how exhilarating it was to find someone whose company you enjoyed. Someone with whom you could talk, laugh, and go places? While you are out connecting with others, be on the lookout for a friend.

Becoming friends takes time and effort. And it requires the willingness to face your fears. After all, there is always the chance that the person with whom you want to be friends doesn't want to be friends with you.

O.K., so there's that chance. Go for it anyway. If you lose, you lose. If you win, you've won something big.

So how do you go from meeting someone you like to becoming friends? You may have to take the first step and call the person.

What do you say when you call? I guess some people might comment on the good connection they felt when they met, and on their desire to become friends. As for me, I've always gone for a more indirect (cowardly?) approach. I call to invite the person to some event. I talk about the activity, noting that I have been planning this for days (not always true) and state that I am going whether or not anyone accompanies me (sometimes true). Then I ask if she would like to come along. By making clear that my participation in the event is not dependent on her, I feel I am giving her a way out. If possible, I try to be flexible on the timing of the activity, as the person may not be able to go on the same weekend or day as I.

Not completely on the up and up? I guess. But it is an approach that works for me.

Even after the initial call, friendships have to be pursued. I usually stick to activity-based calls. I might suggest a movie or taking our kids to the beach or out for ice cream. Sometimes I suggest getting our dogs together.

Something fun and non-threatening.

I know a friendship is forming when I no longer have to give my last name when I call.

One important note. Straight guys often feel uncomfortable trying to make new friends. They worry that new friends will think they are "hitting" on them. So here are a few suggestions. Keep the invites "guy-like." Invite the person to join you and your friends for a game of basketball, a night of watching Monday Night Football, or a game of golf.

Real friends are few, far between, and golden. Don't let your fears stand in your way.

HEAD FOR THE AUTO RACES

The Indy 500 draws hundreds of thousands of spectators a year. And that number accounts only for those seated in the stands or lining the track. Millions more watch on television. Ditto for the Daytona 500. I had to ask. Why are there so many devoted fans? My guess is that we are awe-inspired by the sheer guts it takes to race a formula car two hundred miles an hour around a track. There's also the incredible thrill experienced when a driver crashes and emerges unscathed from a sheer wall of fire. The other appeal: living vicariously so close to the edge of life and death without actually having to step foot in a race car.

So if life starts getting dull, head for the auto races. The Indy 500 happens yearly over Memorial Day weekend, the Daytona 500 in February. However, if the auto race fix hits you in July and patience isn't your strength or traveling is not part of your budget, fine-tune your plans a little. Head to your local drag races for your ration of speed and guts and glory. Check out the souped-up, turbocharged Chevrolets and Fords and the drivers with the wild looks in their eyes. Don't blink, however. Most drag races last ten to fifteen seconds.

RUN

I know a number of people who like to run and a few who love to run. I also know two people who say that a day without a run is a day that is wasted.

Runners claim that running helps reduce their stress. They say they lose themselves in a world of speckled light and inhaled and exhaled breaths. They say that when they finish running, they feel incredibly good.

Some people like to run by themselves, others with buddies. Decide which feels better to you.

Determine when you will run. Choose your days and your time. Some people like to run in the early morning, accompanied only by the birds. Others look forward to running and unwinding at the end of the day. Whatever you choose, stick to it, rain or shine. Don't wait for inspiration.

Some people like the discipline of running, others, the tight abs. Some run a half-mile every morning, some train for marathons. One man I know ran the base of the Grand Canyon three times.

If you feel stuck in a rut, try running. Start off with a short run and increase slowly.

Listen to the music of your breathing.

MEDITATE

Meditation is relaxing. It clears the mind and calms the spirit. It is believed that the results of meditation are long-lasting.

Many people choose a word or phrase to repeat while meditating. This word or phrase helps with focus.

If you are new to meditation, here are some basic tips.

Choose to meditate in a room where there are no distractions. Turn the lights low. Consider lighting some incense or a scented candle. Sit on the floor or in a straight-back chair. Close your eyes and clear your mind. Breathe in and out slowly. Concentrate on your breathing. Repeat the word or phrase you have chosen. When thoughts come to you, push them aside. Sometimes it is helpful to use your hands to push the thoughts away. Try to meditate for at least fifteen minutes at a time. Feel the peace.

FOLLOW THE STOCK MARKET

When I listen to economic gurus talk about stocks and the world economy, it's like listening to Zeus pontificating from the clouds. How do these guys know this stuff? How is Warren Buffett right so often?

My father was a stock market guru of sorts, although on a much, much smaller scale. He was a stock market guru of the everyman variety. My father often tried to teach me how to follow the stock market. I remember there was something called P/E which I never understood. Then there was his stock market philosophy. My father invested in blue chips and utilities. Blue chips are well-known stocks that usually do well, big companies like General Electric and General Motors. Utilities are companies that provide water, power, and electricity to people in a particular area. "Everyone needs utilities," he'd say. More important, utilities pay dividends. Dividends are quarterly payments made to you, the investor, based on the amount of stock you own. "Always reinvest your dividends, Cathy," he'd say. "That way your money grows." My father wasn't one of these buy low and sell high sort of guys. He was a buy low and hold forever sort of guy. His philosophy worked for him.

When I want to feel like a wizard, I follow the stock market. You can too. Go online and look up "stock market." If you want to explore stocks that are hot today (and perhaps gone tomorrow) go to Google and type in phrases like "best stocks" or "great investments." Then wait for the magic of the internet to take you where you want to go. You also can scour the Wall Street Journal for today or tomorrow's darlings. One note of caution. Stocks are risky. Don't invest unless you have money to spare.

GRILL

To grill is to savor the summer. And for some reason, it's more of a guy thing. Even those guys who wouldn't be caught dead sprinkling oregano into a soup, gladly don an apron and grill with joy.

Maybe it's the oversized tools, the big, bulky spatulas that make it O.K. Or maybe it's cooking over an open flame that makes guys feel like they're out in the wild, hunting down antelope.

Whatever the reason, guys like it. On a nice warm day, take out the grill. Invite your friends over. Put some burgers and hot dogs on the grill. As they cook, conduct a sizzle symphony with your spatula. Pop open a Coke or a beer. Put your feet up. Savor the summer.

DO REPAIRS ON YOUR HOUSE

Little lifts our spirits more than being productive. It's as if mom or dad just told us what a great job we did at Little League practice.

While there are lots of ways to be productive, doing a home repair is a big one. Fixing something broken or turning the proverbial ugly duckling into the beautiful swan feels good.

Doing our own home repairs saves money and makes us feel competent and in control. It's like making our own winter coats out of pelts from beavers we ourselves have trapped.

Which home repairs you enjoy has much to do with your sex. Guys are usually into the things that are practical, while women enjoy turning ugly into gorgeous. Translated—guys will find joy in fixing a roof, while women will enjoy tiling the walls surrounding the claw-foot tub.

GO TO THE BEACH

Who doesn't love the beach? The hot sun, the striped umbrellas, the dance of the sea gulls, the sailboats with orange and red spinnakers, the horizon that seems to go on forever.

My favorite beach has a lighthouse in the distance and an old fort. Sometimes, the tides go out so far I can walk almost to the light house. My favorite beach activity is to go at dusk with my kids, spread a blanket, and have a picnic. I don't know why, but when I pack a picnic for the beach, it is always the same: bread, cheese, grapes, Pepsi, homemade chocolate chip cookies, and citronella wrist bands to keep the mosquitoes at bay. My second favorite beach activity is to take my dogs and let them run full speed into the waves after they have played a furious game of tag with the ten-plus other dogs on the beach.

If there is a beach anywhere near you, go and enjoy. Take along a picnic.

ARM CHAIR TRAVEL

Travel is the ultimate good time.

Where would you like to go? New Orleans for the Mardi Gras? Pamplona for the running of the bulls?

Want to climb Mount Everest? Whitewater raft down the Colorado River? Photograph dingoes in Australia or lions in Africa?

Travel is wonderful, but travel is expensive. Seeing the world doesn't have to be.

Go to your library or favorite book store and see what DVDs they have on travel destinations. Or flick on a travel channel. Then grab some chips and salsa, get cozy in your favorite chair, and see the world.

WATCH THE GOOD STUFF ON TELEVISION

I always thought television was a waste of time. Lots of silly sitcoms and stuff I didn't need. Consequently, I never bothered with cable. (I can hear you now. "Don't you ever relax?" To which I say, "Not too easily.") However, over the years, person after person would share with me interesting facts, anecdotes, and stories, then reveal they had gleaned this information from something they had seen on television. One day I saw the proverbial light—maybe I was missing something.

There, I said it.

From there it wasn't too big of a leap to contacting Verizon and having FIOS installed.

Finally, with Verizon's channel guide in hand, I turned on the television. Discovery, National Geographic, Animal Planet, the Travel Channel, NBA TV for the Celtics, and any station airing CSI or Criminal Minds were the channels in which I was interested.

Since I've had television, I have learned some incredible things: Hitler would have died if it hadn't been for one small table leg; energy is released when matter collides (which supports my theory as to what happens when we die); and elephants can paint awesome pictures of other elephants. Also, I have joined a lot of other people in the world and owned up to my fascination with twisted minds. Now tell me this isn't worth fifty dollars a month.

EXPLORE LIFE THROUGH LITERATURE

The Grapes of Wrath, The Executioner's Song, A Death in Belmont, Exodous, Into Thin Air, Loving Frank, The Stranger Beside Me...
Who said sitting still can't be exciting?

COLLECT BASEBALL CARDS

I have a friend who is a crazed baseball card collector. "It's the thrill of the hunt that gets you," he says.

Maybe, but I think there is more.

Maybe it's the nostalgia for the old days. Maybe it's remembering what it was like to be a kid at the ball park, eating hot dogs, and bonding with dad. Maybe it's remembering how much you were going to be just like Babe Ruth. Whatever it is, baseball card collecting has made it to the big leagues.

There are card shops, baseball card shows, and the ever-available eBay where baseball cards, autographed baseballs, and jerseys can be found.

Novice and savvy collectors collect cards, trade them, and sell them. They collect cards of famous players, guys like Mickey Mantle or Willie Mays; rookie cards, cards of players just starting out, before their names are known by third graders and their stats are legends; and error cards, cards on which there have been mistakes such as misspelled names, the wrong color jerseys… The more mint condition the card, the more money it draws. My crazed friend made a hundred dollars on a Carl Yastrzemski rookie card. He said it was "peanuts to what some people make."

WORK ON YOUR CAR

Working on cars is more of a guy thing. I don't know why. Put another way, why do so many guys like changing brake pads while most women like going out for lunch?

When I think of the guys I've known, vehicles come to mind. Max, a nasty but handsome old boyfriend, spent every Saturday on a hard board under his ugly van. Richard, another old boyfriend, thought a guy who didn't change his own oil deserved to spend his weekends watching chick flicks.

Guys say they feel good when they work on their cars. Maybe it's because they have taken care of what is theirs, without asking for outside help.

If you have a car that needs some work, work on it. You will feel good about yourself and save money at the same time.

BUILD SOMETHING

Building something feels good. It builds our confidence. It lets us know we can rely on ourselves.

If you have the skills and the money, build something lasting. If not, build anything. Try your hand at a bird house, a tree house, a bench, a box to store things. If it comes out well, show everyone what you made. If it ends up looking like your eight-year-old cousin made it, say she did.

FISH FOR YOUR DINNER

The best fish I've ever had was caught by a casual friend. While I don't remember the friend, I remember the fish. It was sheepshead. My friend fried the fish in a light beer batter and we ate on the dock overlooking an inlet to the ocean. This was twenty years ago and it is still what I think of when someone asks me about my favorite meal.

There is something incredible about catching your own dinner.

Fishing for your meal makes you feel capable, so at one with nature. And the freshness is guaranteed.

So head for a pier. Or, if you have a friend with a boat, convince her to take you out.

If you ever get the chance to go deep sea fishing, go for it. Pretend you are Ernest Hemingway.

Go. Catch your dinner.

GO CAMPING

I once camped with some friends on the Outer Banks of North Carolina and got eaten by mosquitoes. Another time I camped in the Florida Keys and upon my arrival, was greeted by a group of naked people.

Most people love to camp. They love picking out the camping spots, setting up the tents, making fires, roasting marshmallows, pinpointing the constellations, telling stories, and falling asleep to the sound of the crickets and the frogs.

You can camp in the wild or at a camp site. The wild is probably more beautiful, but you risk running into bears. Once, while on an organized horseback camping trip in Wyoming, I was told not to go outside at night without a cowboy by my side. A cowboy with a rifle. Just in case of grizzlies. I did what I was told and the trip was great.

Camping is relatively cheap and a great way to be one with nature.

Go with friends. The more, the merrier. Avoid the grizzlies. Take mosquito spray.

JOIN A FANTASY BASEBALL/FOOTBALL LEAGUE

My ex-husband was a fantasy baseball fanatic. When we first met, I talked about being a teacher, wanting children, and growing up in New Jersey. He talked about being a teacher and the baseball pitchers he was going to draft for his fantasy baseball team. After being together for six months, I talked about starting a magazine and where we might travel; he talked about the wilderness group he was going to lead for his school and the outfielders he wanted to draft for his fantasy team.

The more comfortable he became with me, the more he talked fantasy baseball. The more he talked, the more I daydreamed. Finally, I told him that I didn't care about his fantasy team. He was heart-broken. I think it did us in.

Fantasy baseball and football team owners are a passionate bunch. They know their stats. They play for money. They clear their schedules and turn off their cell phones for draft day. They form a brotherhood. Don't mess with them.

If you are into baseball or football and don't have a spouse with an aversion to sports, join a fantasy league.

WALK YOUR DOG

He smiles with his tail. He loves you. You can do no wrong.

You owe him.

Walking him is your way of paying him back. So take him for a long walk. Don't hurry him. Let him sniff. In the meantime, enjoy yourself, relax, reflect on the cosmos. And see it as an opportunity. Who knows who might be out there walking her Great Dane?

GO TO A DOG PARK

If you are lucky enough to have a dog park in your town, go there. Dog parks are cool places where dogs play and owners talk. Making small talk is easy because everyone begins their conversations by talking about dogs. If you go often, you likely will see the same people. You might find a friend.

MAKE A PICTURE ALBUM

Think about those most important to you: your family, your friends, your animals. Think about the times you have shared, times that have cracked you up, or made you smile. Think about the experiences that have made you who you are today. Was it that summer at camp when you were bucked off a spotted, white pony seven times and still fell in love with horses? Was it the winter you fell in love with a boy with wild blond hair and a 750 Honda and learned you were a free spirit at heart? Was it the school trip to Manhattan when you realized you wanted to live forever in a city that never slept?

Go through your photos and find these places, these people, these animals. Create an album. Leave the album on your coffee table. Walk through your life.

MAKE A COLLAGE

When my oldest daughter was two, I made a collage of her life. I started with my pregnancy and chose pictures that captured moments throughout her first two years. The pictures were alternately sweet and funny. I laid the pictures out on heavy white poster board and interspersed them with words and phrases I had cut from magazines. After everything was laid out the way I wanted, I glued all the pieces in place. Then I put a coating of shellac on top and let it dry. Later, I framed it in a beautiful beach-colored wood frame. The result was beautiful. And completely personal.

Ask yourself who matters in your life. Then put her in pictures.

CLIMB A MOUNTAIN

In the Boston area where I live, it's something of a hobby to keep track of the Red Sox players' stats and of the mountains you've climbed. It's a status symbol to have climbed Mount Washington. It's a sign of the athletically hopeless to have driven your car up this same mountain.

The fascination with climbing mountains is in the challenge: man pitting himself against the elements, man pushing his body to its limits, man confronting his fears. And the thrill is in accomplishing what he wasn't sure was possible.

If there is a mountain nearby, consider climbing it. But don't be foolish. Make sure your body is up for the job. Take ample supplies, clothing, food, and water. Be prepared for the weather. And follow the advice of your second-grade teacher: go with a buddy.

TRY A NEW FOOD

One of my mother's friends served hamburgers every Saturday, chili every Tuesday, and cold cuts every Friday. One of my daughter's friends eats macaroni and cheese every night. I find myself making the same foods every week: bacon and eggs, hamburgers, chicken, salmon, pizza, and more chicken. And I buy pretty much the same stuff week after week. Then I come home and have nothing I want to eat.

Venture out. Read through the cooking magazines to get ideas. Try out recipes. Do what my youngest daughter does and live and breathe the cooking channels. Explore the ethnic grocery stores in your area. Try your hand at making unusual meals, five-star restaurant meals. Or save your money and go to those small Cuban, Moroccan, or Thai restaurants that are always mobbed. They're packed because they are both good and cheap. Go for lunch. Lunch is cheaper than dinner.

If that's not enough, try octopus or antelope.

GET OUT A CAMERA

You see the world as only you see it, with a perspective that is unique to you. As photographer and photojournalist

Ernst Haas once said, "The camera doesn't make a bit of difference. All cameras can record what you are seeing. But you have to SEE."

So what is it that you see?

Go somewhere special. Set up your camera. Be patient. Wait, watch. Wait for the right lighting, the moment that says it all. Offer your slant to the world.

GO OUT ON A BOAT

Taking a boat into the ocean is a thrilling and humbling experience. Surrounded only by water, you soon realize that you are but one small part of the universe. If you are lucky enough to encounter a school of whales leaping and pirouetting, you will be humbled further, pushed back onto your haunches, in perfect position to be in awe of the natural world.

If you do not own a boat or have a friend willing to take you out on hers, rent a canoe. Get in and paddle slowly. Pay attention to the birds, the trees growing out of nowhere, the lily pads, the uninhabited islands. See nature in its glory.

RIDE A MOTORCYCLE

The wind tickles your face. Your body bends with the curves.

At twenty-two, I explored Europe on the back of a motorcycle. I loved being on that bike. I felt free. If you know someone with a motorcycle, ask to go for a ride. If you are a biker yourself, take your Harley out and cruise.

CLEAN HOUSE

While cleaning is not fun, there is little that feels better than being in a sparkling, clean house. So tackle the job—a room at a time or the whole thing at once. Scrub the floors on your hands and knees. Take a toothbrush to the shower. Wash the curtains. Jazz up the furniture with polish.

Scrub the sink with cleanser. Look around, enjoy, and say, "This is my house."

GET RID OF THINGS

I love to purge. Not food from the fridge, but stuff I don't need. Come spring every year, I have a yard sale. I sell things I've gotten tired of: fabrics that once covered the couch; dog beds on which my dogs refuse to sleep; things I thought I needed but don't (Why did I buy that portable telephone jack system when I don't use my home phone?); presents I have been given but don't like (O. K., I'm not sentimental); things that are ugly. While the yard sales are hard work, I enjoy seeing the stuff I no longer want disappear. Even more, I like stuffing the money I earn into my jeans' pockets.

If yard sales aren't your thing or they sound like too much work, try selling the things you no longer want on eBay. Or donate your goods to charity. Either you will earn money or good karma.

ORGANIZE YOUR HOME

Things are meant to go where they are meant to go.

Dried flowers should not be in with the gas bills. Dog biscuits shouldn't get stuffed in the cabinet with the pasta. Deodorant shouldn't be in with the cleaning supplies.

And clutter makes us crazy. Is there a reason you have five prom dresses? Socks that have no mates? Junk mail that you never read and never will? Coupons from another decade?

Try organizing. It makes you feel good.

While there are lots of ways to organize, I like using baskets. They are cheap and look good, even when full. I use wicker baskets for mail and bushel baskets, the kind farmers use to store fruit, for winter boots.

Go ahead. Organize. And don't forget to throw things out.

REARRANGE YOUR FURNITURE

When people are depressed, they believe things will never change. "Same shit, different day," says one of my clients. While it would be nice to make big changes, big changes can cost. Shaking up things, even a little, makes a difference.

Try rearranging your furniture. Put your couch in a different spot. Take the rug from the bedroom and move it to the dining room. Find a different place for your television. Put your bed against the window. Move the outside in. Grab your outdoor lounge chair, put a cute pillow on it, and make it the focal point of your living room. It may seem like you've moved to new digs.

SCAN THE PAPER FOR JOB OPPORTUNITIES

Many of my clients have been out of work for years. They say they are bored. When I suggest they look for part-time jobs, they say they can't imagine what they would do.

Study the employment section in your local paper to see what's out there. As you read through the list of available jobs, imagine yourself doing the ones that interest you. Visualize yourself pulling into your driveway after a busy shift as a clerk at the book store. Picture yourself tossing off your shoes at home after a four-hour shift transporting patients at the hospital. How does it feel? If it feels good, your next step may be to go for that job.

One note. Some of my clients receive benefits from the government because they have been unable to work. The thought of a part-time job frightens them as they think they will lose their benefits. This is not necessarily true. Check it out before deciding you will be penalized for working.

SCAN THE PAPER FOR GROUPS TO JOIN

Humans are social creatures. We are meant to interact. That's where the brilliance of clubs comes in.

Clubs are groupings of people who share a passion. So begin by asking yourself what it is that you are passionate about.

Is pondering the universe your thing? Hiking? Belly dancing? Are you consumed by depression? Are you preoccupied by the thought of alien encounters?

Then scan the newspaper or internet for clubs in your area.

Find a group. There's one out there for most everybody.

JOIN THE YMCA

Your local YMCA is a gem. For an incredibly cheap price, you get a place to socialize and work out, plus an awesome swimming pool. For a little extra, you get classes—aerobics, yoga, and more. Spend a few months at the "Y." You'll get toned, lose weight, and perhaps, make a friend. Maybe two.

RIDE YOUR BIKE

When I ride a bike, I return to being a kid. I think about what it was like to ride my bike to the rocks, where I would sit cross-legged, eat my snack, and watch the ocean crash into the bay. I think about the summer job I so wanted when I was fourteen. It was a job swimming with dolphins. It's a very good thing I didn't get that job as I'm a lousy swimmer and I have this thing about putting my head under water.

Biking is fun. Ride at your own pace. Go alone, with buddies, or with a group. Ride to the ocean and look for dolphins. Explore back roads. Stop for dinner. Sleep at historic inns.

Make sure your tires have air.

GO FISHING

When I was a child, I would go fishing with my father. We would go on his friend's small motor boat. I remember those days well. "Step on the dock, step on the boat, try not to rock." That was our call to one another. Those days were fun for both my father and me. My father got to spend quality time with his shy, younger daughter and his one really good, male friend. I got to catch eels or blowfish. Blowfish are fish that puff up like balloons when you touch them. Eels are long and slimy and, as I saw things back then, very yucky. We'd always leave the dock early in the morning when the air was full of fog, but it was never long before the sun was blazing and the sky was more yellow than gray. My father always brought along a cooler full of sandwiches, Pepsi, and chocolate. I could eat as much as I wanted.

John, my father's friend and the owner of the boat, would drive the boat slowly. The dark green water would lap its sides. At some point, he'd cut the motor. If I wasn't too busy hanging my feet over the side, I would throw out my line. Neither my father nor I kept the fish we caught, but that wasn't the point. The point was a day on the water and time to be together. Time I still treasure today.

If you are anywhere near the water, go fishing. Join a friend on his boat, cast your rod into the surf, or drop your line from the dock. Take along someone special.

MAKE MONEY CREATIVELY

It is hard to work when your moods are in constant flux. As one of my clients says, "I'll do great for two days. Then I'll wake up and feel awful, so I won't go to work. The next day I'll feel worse, so I'll stay home again. By the third day, when I'm ready to go back to work, I'll find out that I'm fired. I need to make money from home."

Another of my clients says, "For me, it's not the money. It's how I feel when I work. I like to contribute. But I can't work a regular job. I need flexibility."

Many depressed people want to work, but know that they can't always count on their bodies and minds to cooperate. So how do you find a job that allows you to work according to your schedule?

Start by thinking outside of the box. What are your interests? What are your talents? Do you like to fix things? You probably have neighbors who need things repaired. Do you do your own auto repairs? My guess is that you know people who need their engines tuned or brakes replaced. Do you have a passion for dogs? What about dog-sitting for the poodle with bows across the street? Are you a master at whipping up spaghetti and veal piccata? There are people who would love nothing more than to have meals prepared for them.

One very creative woman I know has three young children. She struggles with depression and anxiety. She had a job at an insurance company, but needed more flexibility. As a way to deal with her anxiety, she began painting her nails. She created her own nail designs, first pretty ones, then interesting ones, then complex, intriguing ones. She began buying nail decals, stick-on rhinestones, pearls, dangles. At church on Sunday, teenagers would fawn over her nails. "They're so cool," they'd say. Older women would stop her. "Beautiful nails, my child. I used to have beautiful nails."

My client thought of her grandmother and how her grandmother so loved looking beautiful. She remembered how she had painted her grandmother's nails one Christmas. "Nanny" had looked so regal. It turned out to be her grandmother's last Christmas.

An idea brewed.

"I'm going to get certified in nails. I'll create a portfolio of my designs. I'm going to provide a mobile service. I'll go around to assisted living places, nursing homes, fairs… I won't charge much. I'll make my own schedule. I'll go when I can. It will be fun. I'll make people happy. And I'll be home more with the kids."

"Brilliant," I said. "Brilliant idea."

Believe in you.

PERFORM AN ACT OF KINDNESS

You have heard it said and it's true. Giving is better than receiving. Do something nice just for the sake of doing it. Plant flowers for your aunt. Bring out your neighbor's trash. Sneak over to your friend's house early on Easter morning and leave a big, stuffed Easter bunny for her daughter. Sign it, "Love, Mr. Bunny." Wrap a Christmas present and leave it, anonymously, on the doorstep of someone who has been having a hard year. Make treats for your neighborhood animals. Collect teddy bears and take them to a homeless shelter.

WRITE A LETTER OF THANKS TO SOMEONE WHO HAS MADE A DIFFERENCE IN YOUR LIFE

Years ago I read something that so impressed me, I still think of it today. While on a navy ship, a sailor, who later became a very famous author, wrote to five individuals who he believed had had a profound impact on his life. Some of these were folks he knew well, others were people he barely knew. One was a writer whose inspiring story he had learned through an article in a national newspaper. However, all of these individuals had helped shape the sailor's beliefs and character. Between shifts swabbing the deck, he took the time to thank them.

Is there someone in your life you would like to thank? Someone who has helped make you the person you are today? Someone who has loved you enough to stand in your way when doing so was just what you needed? Someone who helped you move on from your mistakes?

Have you ever thanked her? Have you ever told him what he meant to you?

Life is short. Thank her while you can.

PLANT FLOWERS

If reincarnation exists, I am putting in my order. I want to come back as 1) a person, 2) a golden retriever, 3) a wild mustang, 4) a sea gull, 5) a sunflower.

"But sunflowers don't last very long," you say.

You're right. But they are so beautiful.

You can have a garden wherever you live. If you are lucky enough to have a yard, your choices are endless. I love to plant flowers that dazzle and grow tall—morning glory, clematis, and you guessed it, sunflowers.

If you're an apartment dweller, go for window boxes. Pansies, violas, petunias, and impatiens are small, colorful, and beautiful.

Go ahead, plant some flowers. Make yourself smile.

GROW YOUR OWN VEGETABLES

Fresh grown tomatoes have a taste all their own. The same is true for lettuce and other vegetables right out of the garden. Add some olive oil and a dash of oregano and imagine you are in your courtyard in Tuscany. To grow your own vegetables, you need only an area of garden or some plant containers, some small vegetable plants, and a stake or tomato cage to hold up the vegetables. Plant when there is no danger of frost. Then feast.

GO TO A FLEA MARKET

In my life, going to the flea market is a Sunday morning tradition. I love awakening on a Sunday morning when the sun is bright, and heading out, chocolate frosted donut in-hand, to a nearby, five-acre field filled with table after table of flea market treasures. While I have brought home many treasures, my favorite is a light blue, hand-painted window with a background of pond lilies.

My flea market also has great popcorn.

No two flea markets are exactly alike. The one I enjoy is known for furniture and antiques. A flea market in a nearby state sells only pocketbooks and jewelry.

To get the dirt on the markets around you, go to the source: your bargain-hunting female friends.

GO SOMEWHERE AND HAVE A PICNIC

Summer and picnics go together. Think of your favorite place—the place you can see with your eyes closed. Go there and have a picnic. For me, it is the beach at dusk. I always bring my entourage of animate beings—kids, friends, dogs (if allowed); things—blankets, sweatshirts, citronella wrist bands; and food—curried chicken salad, French bread, grapes, bakery-bought chocolate chip cookies, and Pepsi. I didn't say healthy, I said picnic.

LEARN ANOTHER LANGUAGE

In high school I studied French. I didn't do very well.

The one and only time I have been to France, I tried to use the language I never had mastered.

We were in Arles, France.

My children and I noticed that a bull fight was being held. We were interested, but being animal lovers, we wanted to make sure that the bulls were not going to be killed.

I approached the man at the booth and asked, in what I thought was proper French, if the bulls were going to be hurt.

"No, madam," I heard, followed by something I interpreted as, "We are very gentle with our animals."

Well, who knows what I asked, because gentle they were not.

What language would you like to learn? Spanish? Chinese? Arabic?

Call your local community college or university to find out what's being offered. Then go take a course.

CHAPTER TEN

HURDLES

DEPRESSED PEOPLE OFTEN RESIST SUGGESTIONS. It is not because they are being difficult. It is because they believe change is impossible. Depression has been their bed partner for too long.

DON'T SHOOT YOURSELF IN THE FOOT

One of my clients is a very personable man in his early sixties. A physical disability prevents him from standing for long. Unfortunately, this forced him to give up his job as a baker. It was a job he loved.

Having lived on disability for seven years now, my client is accustomed to money problems. The fourth week of every month is tough: nightly dinners of macaroni and cheese or hot dogs and beans. He seldom goes out as he does not have the money to do so. He is very isolated and depressed. He had a girlfriend of sorts, but ended the relationship because he could not afford to take her anywhere. "I couldn't even take her to McDonald's," he said.

I suggest to my client that he get a part-time job.

"I can't stand," he says.

"So sit," I say. "You've got a great personality."

"No," he says. "Nobody wants me to sit. Besides, if I work, I'll lose my benefits."

I explain that people are allowed to make some money while receiving benefits.

"No," he says. "If I make money, my rent will go up. And my food stamps will go down. I'll end up working for nothing."

I disagree. "You'll end up with more money than you have now. Plus, you'll be out with people. It'll be social. You'll like it."

"No," he says "Plus, some days I don't want to get up."

"I know," I say. "But remember, the best way to beat depression is to do some of what you don't want to do."

"No," he says. "It won't work."

"How do you know if you don't try?"

CHRONIC PAIN

Many of the depressed clients with whom I work are in chronic pain. Some are in pain from car accidents, others from work-related injuries, still others from conditions they have had since childhood.

Some chronic pain can be successfully treated, other pain not so, as the catalyst for the pain is unknown or the pain is the result of a condition that does not respond well to treatment.

I can't imagine what it is like to live with chronic pain, to awaken every day and go to bed every evening with the body aching, throbbing, and screaming. I'm sure it is horrible.

But this I know. You have only one life to live. You have to do everything possible to tolerate your pain. You have to fight your pain as if you were fighting off a crazed and half-starved bear. It's your life or his.

My sister has done an admirable job of living with pain. It has not been easy. She suffers from crippling scoliosis. She has had two major surgeries and has metal rods in both her chest and back. Sometimes, she's in so much pain, she can do little but cry. But she seldom gives in. She has found a way to coexist with her pain, this roommate she never wanted. She has created a way to make money from home. This allows her down time when she needs it.

She refuses to be confined to her home. She goes out often, but always tries to keep walking to a minimum. She sits when she needs to, finding chairs in stores or benches along the way. If the amount of walking is going to be too great, she takes along her wheelchair. She could be too proud and refuse the wheelchair, but she's smarter than that. She travels, although staying at home would be easier. "I'm not going to miss out on seeing the world," she says. Soon she is going to Egypt to see the pyramids. "If I'm in pain, so be it," she says. "But I'm going to see them." She never lifts. She has cortisone shots when she needs them. She stays on medication which keeps the worst of her pain at bay, even though the medications have side effects. She sleeps more than she wants to. She lives by the motto that life is short and meant to be lived fully. She battles her pain daily.

One of my clients has painful fibromyalgia. She goes to a pain clinic and finds massage therapy helpful. She eats fruits, vegetables, and lean meats only, and walks a mile or more a day. She works part-time as a nanny, because she loves kids. Lifting the children is difficult, but she does so anyway. On good days, she swings them around and wrestles with them. On really good days, she camps out with them in the woods in a fort that she and they built. On bad days, she stays home and sleeps.

A man I know suffers from chronic shoulder pain from an injury he sustained. He was an artist, but had to give it up. "Constantly lifting my brush was too much," he said. "Realizing I couldn't give up the creativity, I decided to try my hand at writing. It's different," he says. "I'm not quite used to it, but I like it. However, sometimes, I have to get someone else to type for me." After three years, he has finished his first draft of a novel.

What helps with chronic pain is a question with few easy answers.

Some find antidepressants helpful. This is because the brain pathways that handle the reception of pain rely on some of the same neurotransmitters that are involved with mood. Also, as pain has so many down sides, chronic sufferers often are depressed. And of course, antidepressants help with depression. Talk to your doctor to see if antidepressants are an option.

Stress reduction techniques such as progressive muscle relaxation, hypnosis, meditation, visualization, and journaling can help take off pain's jagged edge.

Working with a physical therapist is helpful as they are trained to create exercise plans specifically designed for particular areas of pain.

Ditto for working with a psychiatric therapist. As these therapists are trained to help people consider different perspectives, a therapist can help pain sufferers broaden the possibilities of life with chronic discomfort.

Many pain sufferers say pain medication is needed to smooth the raw edges. Doctors routinely prescribe non-addictive medications to help. But often these don't do the trick. This leads people to seek out stronger pain medication.

But here's the rub. Many of the stronger pain medications are narcotics and many doctors are hesitant to prescribe them, for fear the patient will abuse them or become addicted.

If you have tried alternative approaches and feel that you cannot function without narcotic pain medication, you are going to have to be a strong advocate for yourself. Drug addiction is awful, but taking a medication to moderate your pain is responsible. However, you are going to have to convince your doctor that you will be responsible. While you may feel insulted by your doctor's hesitancy in prescribing these medications, you cannot take it personally. Realize that she needs to know that you have exhausted your other alternatives and that you will be a responsible patient. No matter how sincere you are, you have to remain vigilant. Narcotics are slippery.

Participating in a group with other pain sufferers is a good idea. Not only will you find others who understand what you are going through, but you will be able to share ideas about pain management and treatments. And the moral support can be invaluable. Only people who live through daily pain understand what it is like. Look in your local newspaper or call your area hospital to see if there is such a group. If not, consider starting one by advertising in your area newspaper.

I recently heard a wonderful story.

One of my college friends has rheumatoid arthritis. Over the years, her arthritis has spread and it is now in her lungs. She has to use oxygen and cannot walk far.

She is on the list for a lung transplant. She is much too young for this.

She lives in Florida.

Recently, one of her close friends invited her to his wedding in Napa Valley, California. He had invited only his ten best friends. My friend was one.

My friend replied that she would attend even if she had to be flown to California on a stretcher.

Fortunately, a stretcher wasn't needed.

She and all the groom's friends spent a week in California. My friend had to use a wheel chair for many of the activities. The highlight of the week was a balloon ride at dawn over Napa Valley. My friend agreed to go along and ride in the chaser car while the others went in the balloon.

When they arrived at the balloon site, my friend had to be pushed in a wheel chair. The balloon was there in all its glory. So was the chaser car. My friend looked at the balloon. You only get one shot at this life, she thought.

Her friends were already in the balloon. She asked the balloon handlers if they would lift her into the balloon. They did.

She and the groom's other friends floated over the valley. The sun shone. They could see everything.

She said it was an incredible once-in-a-lifetime, magnificent experience.

I say a woman this brave deserves magnificence.

CHAPTER ELEVEN
TYING IT ALL TOGETHER

NOW THAT YOU HAVE FINISHED reading the book, it is time to take three deep breaths and put the mood-changing plan into action. But first, there are several preliminary steps.

Step number one is to make several copies of the mood-changing daily calendar. Tack at least two copies of the calendar onto your walls in very visible spots. Consider the calendar your most essential tool. The calendar spells out everything you need to do to smash your depression.

Step number two is to make copies of all forms. The form you will be using most often is the "Automatic Thought Form." Make enough copies of this form to last through week one. Next week, you can make more. Keep all of your forms together in one folder.

Next is to determine how, when, and where you will carry out each activity.

Brainstorm with your family and friends for ideas on this. Consider the pros and cons of the different possibilities. Then, make your decisions and write them down.

Your final step is to tell yourself that you can do this. And you can. Yes, it will be work and yes, some of it will be hard. But by the end, you will be well on your way to becoming the person you have always wanted to become.

O.K., YOU'RE READY

Give yourself tremendous credit. You have been honest and acknowledged that you have a problem. You have depression. You have admitted that you have not done enough about it. You have dealt with your anger, cursed out the universe. Reluctantly, you have let your wishful thinking go and accepted that tackling depression takes work. You have read this book when you would have preferred to watch television. Now you are ready to act.

Good for you.

If you follow the plan, you will start feeling better. In two months, you will have less difficulty getting up in the morning. In five months, you may surprise yourself by having a really nice thought about…you. In nine months, you will find that you are starting to live a life that seems… kind of awesome.

But you have to keep up with the plan indefinitely. You are feeling better because you have changed your behaviors and altered how you think about yourself. Remember what I said before. Depression is like a grizzly bear. If you drop your depression-fighting activities like so much food, the grizzly will find you.

So start the plan. Grab your life with your freckled arms in a big, old hug and don't let go. Hold on tight. Say, "I've got one life to live and I'm going for it." Say, "I'm worth it."

You can do it.

RESOURCES

American Academy of Child and Adolescent Psychiatry
www.aacap.org
American Psychological Association (APA)
www.apa.org
Beating Depression and Anxiety
www.beatingdepressionandanxiety.com
Depression and Bipolar Support Alliance (DBSA)
www.dbsalliance.org
Mental Health America
www.mentalhealthamerica.net
National Alliance on Mental Illness (NAMI)
www.nami.org
National Institute of Mental Health
www.nimh.nih.gov
Stress, Anxiety and Depression Resource Center
www.stress-anxiety-depression.org

REFERENCES

"Avoiding Depression: Sleeping in Dark Room May Help." LiveScience. *17 Nov. 2010.* http://www.livescience.com/9004-avoiding-depression-sleeping-dark-room.html.

Burns, David D. *Feeling Good: The New Mood Therapy.* New York: Morrow, 1980.

Clarke, Jacqueline, and Joanna Farrow. *Mediterranean Food of the Sun.* London: Hermes House, 2009.

Cloutier, Marissa, and Eve Adamson. *The Mediterranean Diet.* New York: Harper/Harper Collins, 2001.

Hibbeln, J. "Fish Consumption and Major Depression." *The Lancet* 351.9110 (1998): 1213.

Hibbeln, Joseph R., John M. Davis, Colin Steer, Pauline Emmett, Imogen Rogers, Cathy Williams, and Jean Golding. "Maternal Seafood Consumption in Pregnancy and Neurodevelopmental Outcomes in Childhood (ALSPAC Study): an Observational Cohort Study." *The Lancet* 369.9561 (2007): 578-85.

Lanou, Amy Joy., and Michael Castleman. *Building Bone Vitality: A Revolutionary Diet Plan to Prevent Bone Loss and Reverse Osteoporosis.* New York: McGraw-Hill, 2009.

Sánchez-Villegas, A., P. Henríquez, M. Bes-Rastrollo, and J. Doreste. "Mediterranean Diet and Depression." *Public Health Nutrition* 9.8A (2006).

Stoll, Andrew L. *The Omega-3 Connection: The Groundbreaking Omega-3 Antidepression Diet and Brain Program.* New York: Simon & Schuster, 2001.

Walker, Morton. *The Power of Color.* Garden City Park, NY: Avery Publishing Group, 1991.

ABOUT THE AUTHOR

Cathy Goldstein Mullin is a therapist on the North Shore of Boston. She has a private practice where she sees children, adolescents, and adults, many of whom struggle with depression. She is also a staff therapist at a large teaching hospital. For the last several years, she has led workshops and given talks on her areas of expertise. *If I Could Just Snap Out of It, Don't You Think I Would? A Nine-Month Plan for Smashing Your Depression* is her first book. She is presently at work on another book, tentatively titled *The Wicked Sisters Who Live in the Pit: Taming the Beasts of Your Anxiety*. In 2009, she launched a website offering information and treatment for anxiety and depressive disorders.

Contact information for Cathy Goldstein Mullin:
email: cathygoldsteinmullin@hotmail.com or cgsierra@hotmail.com;
website: www.beatingdepressionandanxiety.com